Keto Diet for Beginners: The Ultimate Meal Plan & Eating Out Guide for Effective Low Carb Weight Loss & Healthy Living Using Ketosis

This book contains 2 manuscripts:

Keto Diet on the Go: *Your Ultimate Guide to Low-Carb Friendly Options at America's Favorite Restaurants*

Keto Meal Prep: *How to Save $100 and 4 Hours A Week by Batch Cooking*

By Jason Michaels

Table of Contents

Keto Diet on The Go
Chapter 1: Keto Options: Well-Known Chain Restaurants..9
Chapter 2: Keto Options at Generic Non-Chain/Mom & Pop Restaurants..81
Chapter 3: Keto Options at Convenience Stores & Gas Stations.. 90
Chapter 4: Keto Options: Low Carb Alcoholic & Coffee Beverages..95
Chapter 5: Keto Imposters &"Contraband"...............100
Chapter 6: Helpful Tips & Guidelines........................106
Conclusion...114

Keto Meal Prep
Introduction... 117
Chapter 1: Brief Overview of the Keto Diet............... 119

    Fat Torch Versus Sugar Burner.......................... 119
    Keto Diet Benefits... 120
    Foods to Avoid... 121
    Food to Embrace..122

Chapter 2: Why You Should Be Meal Prepping.......... 123

    What is Meal Prepping?.....................................123
    Reasons Why You Should Be Meal Prepping.....124

Chapter 3: How to Avoid the 10 Most Common Meal Prep Mistakes.. 128
Chapter 4: Delicious Keto Recipes............................. 135

> Breakfast Recipes..136
> Lunch Recipes... 155
> Mason Jar Recipes...172
> Dinner Recipes.. 185
> Dessert Recipes...207
> Fat Bomb Recipes..214
> Rice Alternatives... 230

Emergency Keto Meals at Popular Fast Food Chains 232
Chapter 5: Methods to Properly Store Food............. 235
Chapter 6: Meal Prep Kitchen Essentials................... 239

© Copyright 2018 by Jason Michaels - All rights reserved.

The following eBook is reproduced below with the goal of providing information that is as accurate and reliable as possible. Regardless, purchasing this eBook can be seen as consent to the fact that both the publisher and the author of this book are in no way experts on the topics discussed within and that any recommendations or suggestions that are made herein are for entertainment purposes only. Professionals should be consulted as needed prior to undertaking any of the action endorsed herein.

This declaration is deemed fair and valid by both the American Bar Association and the Committee of Publishers Association and is legally binding throughout the United States.

Furthermore, the transmission, duplication or reproduction of any of the following work including specific information will be considered an illegal act irrespective of if it is done electronically or in print. This extends to creating a secondary or tertiary copy of the work or a recorded copy and is only allowed with express written consent from the Publisher. All additional right reserved.

The information in the following pages is broadly considered to be a truthful and accurate account of facts and as such any inattention, use or misuse of the information in question by the reader will render any resulting actions solely under their purview. There are no scenarios in which the publisher or the original author of this work can be in any fashion deemed liable for any hardship or damages that may befall them after undertaking information described herein.

Additionally, the information in the following pages is intended only for informational purposes and should thus be thought of as universal. As befitting its nature, it is presented without assurance regarding its prolonged validity or interim quality. Trademarks that are mentioned are done without written consent and can in no way be considered an endorsement from the trademark holder.

Introduction

You've conquered the first step by getting your body into ketosis. One of the many perks of this eating lifestyle is its sustainability. There are so many good foods that you can eat while in ketosis that will keep you satisfied and you won't even miss the bread! However, it's one thing to stick to the plan when you're doing your own meal prep. It's a whole new ballgame when you take your new eating habits out into the world. There are a few things you can do before reaching the restaurant of choice that will hopefully make the process a bit easier.

First, when possible, try not go out to eat on an empty stomach. If you're already somewhat satisfied you'll be able to resist temptations that much better. Even if you chug a glass of room temperature water before you leave, your stomach will feel more full.

If you've planned ahead, do your research before getting to the restaurant. Almost every chain restaurant has its full menu publically available. Decide which direction you want to take your meal and any off-menu modifications you might want to make. That way, when it comes time to order you'll know exactly what you want and how many carbs it will cost you.

Pack food ahead of time for trips. That will make you less likely to splurge on carby snacks at the gas station or airport.

Finally, don't stress out! It's understandable that asking for off-menu items can be a bit intimidating. There is always the risk that your dining companion might not understand or the order might arrive incorrect or incomplete. And that's okay! Because it will happen, on occasion, but at the end of the day, you are the one that matters.

So get ready to dive into the low-carb faction of the restaurant world. Bon appetit!

Side Note: net carbs are calculated by subtracting total fiber from total carbs

There are plenty of books on this subject on the market, thanks again for choosing this one! Every effort was made to ensure it is full of as much useful information as possible, please enjoy!

Chapter 1: Keto Options: Well-Known Chain Restaurants

Eating out, in general, can make it difficult to maintain dieting goals. Sticking to a diet at our favorite, well-known restaurants can up the challenge considerably. Thankfully, healthier trends in food preparation and low-carb options made available have made an appearance in a wide variety of our better-known chains.

Denny's

Good ol' Denny's; comforting, easy on the pocketbook, and they're always open! Resisting favorites could be difficult at this family favorite sit-down restaurant, but where there is a will, there is a way. And thankfully, there are quite a few ways to make these potentially carb-loaded meals much more keto friendly. Many of these low-carb options are appropriate for breakfast, lunch, or dinner.

T-Bone Steak & Eggs: This is about as perfect for low-carb eating as you can get...if all you were served was the steak and the eggs. Forgoing sides is a sacrifice that must be made, so to keep this favorite keto friendly, leave out extras such as toast and hash browns and it comes to about 1g net carbs.

Grand Slam (build-your-own): The Grand Slam is definitely on the favorites list. Here is a list of ingredients you could use to customize it to your liking and diet goals:

Bacon (2 strips= 1g net carbs), turkey bacon (2 strips= 1g net carbs), sausage (2 links= 0g net carbs), eggs (2= 1g net carbs), egg whites (2= 1g net carbs), grilled ham (3oz. slice= 3g net carbs), gouda-apple chicken sausage (1 link= 2g net carbs).

Use this list to mix and match to your liking, staying away from the pancakes, of course.

Favorite Omelettes: Denny's offers a variety of omelettes that are typically Keto friendly as they are, just be sure to leave out the "carby" sides:

Ham & Cheese Omelette: 7g net carbs

Ultimate Omelette®: 8g net carbs

Loaded Veggie Omelette: 7g net carbs

Philly Cheese-steak Omelette: 11g net carbs

Skillets: Denny's skillets are another great option, just be sure to get them without the potatoes. There was no data available on the exact net carbs on the skillets, but as long as they are potato free they should all fall below 10g:

Fit Fare® Veggie Skillet

Crazy Spicy Skillet (option to add eggs)

Supreme Skillet (option to add eggs)

Wild Alaska Salmon Skillet

Santa Fe Skillet (option to add eggs)

Salads & Sides: You can never go wrong with a salad! Well, I guess technically you can, but as long as you stick to these low-carb options you'll be on the right track:

Prime Rib Cobb Salad (no dressing): 12g net carbs

Veggies with Ranch Dip: 3g net carbs

Avocado Chicken Caesar Salad (16 oz.): 8g net carbs

Tilapia Ranchero (no bread): 3g net carbs

T-Bone Steak (no bread): 5g net carbs

Sirloin Steak (no bread): 3g net carbs

Burgers/Sandwiches: None of these options will start as low-carb because of the bread and some of the condiments. To make these sandwiches keto friendly, order without the bread, possibly in a lettuce wrap, avoid sugary condiments such as BBQ sauce and ketchup, and skip the fries or substitute with cut veggies. Try to limit or avoid fruit as sides.

Condiments: Condiment options will probably be very similar across the board at any restaurant, but here are some specific to Denny's:

Ranch Dressing (1.5oz): 1g net carbs

Buffalo Sauce (2oz): 2g net carbs

Blue Cheese Dressing (1.5oz): 3g net carbs

Caesar Dressing (1.5oz): 0g net carbs

Italian Dressing (Fat free, 1.5oz): 4g net carbs

Sour Cream (1.5oz): 2g net carbs

IHOP

IHOP options will be very similar to Denny's and the same rules for entrees, sandwiches and burgers will apply: skip the bread, potatoes, and sweet condiments. Some of the main menu, however, can be ordered with little to no alterations.

Omelettes: Something to keep in mind; some of the research has discovered that IHOP puts pancake batter in their eggs when they make the omelettes, which obviously has an effect on the net carbs. Be sure to request real eggs when ordering.

Colorado Omelette: 13g net carbs

Avocado, Bacon, Cheese Omelette: 5g net carbs

Corned Beef Hash & Cheese Omelette: 20g net carbs

Bacon Temptation Omelette: 10g net carbs

Bacon, Sausage, and Eggs: When in doubt, keep it simple...good ol' bacon and eggs! Eggs (basic serving size is usually 2) can be fried, poached, scrambled, or boiled and they will contain about 1-2g net carbs. Sausage or bacon are usually about 1g net carbs for an order. Order just bacon and/or sausage and eggs (no sides) and you'll have a fulfilling meal that will keep you in ketosis.

Salads/Dressings: As with any salad, the danger is most often in the dressing, both the type and the quantity.

Grilled Chicken Cobb: 10g net carbs (without the dressing)

House Salad: 3g net carbs (without the dressing)

Caesar Salad (side, 12g net carbs, without the dressing)

The dressings are what launch the net carbs upward, so take care when ordering! Get the dressing on the side to help keep the carb load down.

Waffle House

Yet another diner style, comforting, carb-laden restaurant. And still, there are plenty of low carb options to choose from.

Omelettes: Avoid sides (toast, hash browns, etc.).

Ham & Cheese Omelette: 10g net carbs

Fiesta Omelette: 7g net carbs

Cheese-steak Omelette: 6g net carbs

Breakfast Staples

Bacon (3 slices): 0g net carbs

Country Ham (1 slice): 0g net carbs

Sausage (2 patties): 0g net carbs

Eggs w/ Cheese (2 eggs, equivalent of 1 slice of cheese): 1g net carbs

Sausage Egg & Cheese Wrap: 25g Net Carbs

Meat: Most meat choices, without any kind of sauce or gravy, are going to be 0g net carbs.

Burgers/Sandwiches: Same rule applies as before; skip the bread, sweet condiments, and fries. Maybe try adding a fried egg on top of a bunless burger to make it more interesting.

California Pizza Kitchen

In order to stay low carb at California Pizza Kitchen, you may have to forgo the pizza. However, their low carb options are still very good and will provide a fulfilling meal while remaining in ketosis.

Salads

Italian Chopped Salad (half portion): 9g net carbs

Classic Caesar Salad (full portion): 12g net carbs

Roasted Veggie & Grilled Shrimp Salad (half portion): 17g net carbs

California Cobb Salad (full portion, including ranch dressing): 13g net carbs

Appetizers/Entrees

Lettuce Wraps (order with chicken or shrimp or both!)

Grilled Chicken Chimichurri: 13g net carbs

Fire-Roasted Chile Relleno: 20g net carbs

Grilled Chicken Breast (no sauces/sides): 0g net carbs

Power Bowls: These are definitely healthier options; for keto diets, they may still need to be tweaked just a bit. No net carb info available, but here are some suggestions to make sure these bowls stay keto friendly:

Shanghai Power Bowl: This meal comes with shrimp and a variety of vegetables such as cauliflower, baby broccoli, carrots, and zucchini. It also includes Forbidden Rice® and house made Shanghai sauce, both of which should probably be held off (or at least on the side) to keep the carbs down.

Santa Fe Bowl: This bowl includes lime chicken, sweet corn, tomatoes, black beans, avocado, poblano peppers, red cabbage, and toasted pepitas on top of spinach and cilantro farr0. It is served with CPK's house made ranch. To keep this bowl keto friendly, it would be best to skip the corn and ask for dressing on the side.

Banh Mi Bowl: This bowl consists of baby kale, quinoa, mint, and cilantro topped by grilled chicken, radishes, watermelon, avocado, carrots, bean sprouts, cucumbers, scallions, and sesame seeds. It comes with CPK's chili and lime vinaigrette and Serrano peppers. While quinoa is very healthy, it is also very high in protein. Unused protein is broken down into sugar and stored as fat.

Cauliflower Crust: CPK has recently come out with a cauliflower crust, reportedly consisting of cauliflower, rice flour, mozzarella, and some spices and herbs. This is great news for vegetarians but perhaps not so much for keto and low-carb as one slice is 90 calories and has 14g net carbs. It might be best to stick with non-pizza meals in order to remain in ketosis.

Chili's

Chili's actually has a section in their menu called "Guiltless Grills". Some items on this part of the menu may be a bit too high in starch, which bumps net carbs up to 50g and over. However, there are a few specific dishes that are perfect for the keto diet (all listed not including the sides that come with some of the entrees).

Guiltless Grills & Other Main Dishes

Guiltless Cedar Plank Tilapia: Seasoned tilapia fillet with Chili's house made pico de gallo and served on a cedar plank; 3g net carbs.

Guiltless Grilled Salmon: 8oz of salmon seasoned and seared; 5g net carbs.

Salmon with Garlic and Herbs: 1g net carbs

Guiltless Carne Asada Steak Sirloin: The meat is seasoned and flame grilled and also comes with the house made pico de gallo; 5g net carbs.

Spicy Garlic & Lime Grilled Shrimp: 7g net carbs

Pepper Pals Grilled Chicken Platter (on the kids' menu): 4g net carbs

Chili's Classic Sirloins: 1g net carbs

Starters

Caesar Salad (side portion, no croutons!): approximately 6g net carbs

Triple Dipper Wings over Buffalo with Blue Cheese: 2g net carbs

Cup Chicken Enchilada: 8g net carbs

Terlinga Chili (cup): 7g net carbs

Lunch Combo House Salad (Hold the dressing): 9g net carbs

Extras/Sides

Dressings: Blue Cheese, Avocado Ranch, and Caesar

Avocado Slices

Side of Guacamole (small)

Sautéed Mushrooms

All Cheeses

Sour Cream

Steamed Broccoli

Cut veggies (celery, carrots)

Applebee's

Applebee's also has a low carb section on their menu, making it much easier to pick keto friendly meals.

Starters

Double Crunch Bone-In Wings (either with blue cheese or ranch dressing): 13g net carbs

Double Crunch Bone-In Wings (no sauce or dressing): 10g net carbs

Double Crunch Bone-In Wings (classic Buffalo): 13g net carbs

Main Dishes (from the grill)

Doubled-Glazed Baby Back Ribs (both half rack and full rack, no sauce): 0g net carbs

Fire-Grilled Shrimp Skewer: 1g net carbs

12oz Top Sirloin (Butcher's Reserve): 0g net carbs

USDA Top Sirloin 6oz: 1g net carbs

USDA Top Sirloin 8oz: 2g net carbs

Shrimp 'N Parmesan Sirloin: 5g net carbs

Grilled Chicken Breast: 0g net carbs

Lunch Dishes

Thai Shrimp Salad: 12g net carbs

Tomato Basil Soup (cup): 13g net carbs

Southwest Black Bean Soup (cup): 12g net carbs

Grilled Chicken Caesar Salad (no croutons!): 8g net carbs

House Salads: Some of these salads are a bit higher in the carb range than you might want, especially if you plan on getting an entrée as well. Be mindful of dressing choice/quantity and leave off extras such as croutons, chips, fruit, and nuts.

House Salad w/ Buttermilk Ranch: 13g net carbs
House Salad w/ Garlic Caesar: 13g net carbs

House Salad w/ Blue Cheese: 13g net carbs

House Salad w/ Lemon Olive Oil Vinaigrette: 10g net carbs

House Salad w/ Mexi Ranch: 13g net carbs

House Salad w/ Italian: 15g net carbs

House Salad w/ Green Goddess: 12g net carbs

Small Caesar: 9g net carbs

Green Goddess Wedge Salad: 9g net carbs

House Salad (no dressing): 10g net carbs

Sides

Garlicky Green Beans w/ Bacon: 7g net carbs

Fire-Grilled Veggies: 6g net carbs

Steamed Broccoli: 3g net carbs

Wendy's

As with other restaurants serving burger and sandwiches, all of these low-carb options from Wendy's are bunless.

Burger & Meat Options (no condiments or toppings)

Jr. Hamburger Patty: 0g net carbs

Single Hamburger Patty: 0g net carbs

Grilled Chicken Breast: 3g net carbs

Applewood Smoked Bacon (1 strip): 0g net carbs

Toppings/Condiments: The stand-alone meat options are very low in net carbs. Which means you can add to your order as you keep track of the carb count in these condiments and toppings.

Cheeses: American 1 slice= 1g net carbs, Asiago 1 slice= 1g net carbs, cheddar 1 slice= 0g net carbs, shredded cheddar= 1g net carbs, cheddar cheese sauce= 1g net carbs

Mayonnaise: 0g net carbs

Mustard: 0g net carbs

Pickles, onions, and iceberg lettuce: all 0g net carbs

Tomato: 1 slice= 1g net carbs

Tartar Sauce: 0g net carbs

Salads

Garden Salad (without dressing and croutons): 5g net carbs

Caesar Salad (without dressing and croutons): 4g net carbs

Sauces/Dressing

Ranch: 2g net carbs

Buttermilk Ranch (dipping sauce): 2g net carbs

Light Ranch: 2g net carbs

Italian: 4g net carbs

Lemon Garlic Caesar: 2g net carbs

Thousand Island: 5g net carbs

Meal Pairing Ideas: Now that we know individual options, we can mix and match meals. These won't necessarily have a spot on the actual menu, but they d0 fulfill the requirements for low-carb options.

Three Double-Stack Cheeseburgers (dry, no bun) with pickles, wrapped in lettuce: 3g net carbs

Grilled Chicken (dry, no bun), garden side salad w/ ranch, Diet Coke: 7g net carbs

Two Jr. Bacon Cheeseburgers (dry, no bun) with Caesar salad (no dressing or croutons), and small Minute Maid Lemonade: 11g net carbs

Triple Baconator (dry, no bun) mayo on the side, bottle of water: 3g net carbs

KFC

Everything about KFC says "comfort food". There is nothing specifically on the menu labeled as low-carb, but if KFC is absolutely the last option for a meal, there is a smart way to order to stay on the keto diet.

Meal Ideas

There aren't a lot of chicken options that will stick with the keto diet, so the Kentucky Grilled Chicken Breast is probably the only way to go:

Two Kentucky Grilled Chicken Breasts with a small side of green beans and maybe a side of creamy buffalo dip comes to about 6g net carbs.

Sides

Caesar Salad (no dressing): 1g net carbs

Side Salad (no dressing): 1g net carbs

Sauce

Creamy Buffalo: 2g net carbs

Buttermilk Ranch: 2g net carbs

Dressing

Marzetti Light Italian: 2g net carbs

KFC Creamy Parmesan Caesar: 4g net carbs

Heinz Buttermilk Ranch: 1g net carbs

McDonald's

All of the McDonald's low-carb options take out the bun or bread (biscuit, muffins) and have no ketchup included. The buns alone on the burgers account for more than ¾ of the carb count listed on the nutrition facts!

Breakfast: There really aren't a whole lot of low-carb options for breakfast since most of their famous breakfast options include muffins, biscuits, and/or syrup.

Modified Egg McMuffin: take out the muffin, keep the egg, American cheese, and ham or sausage and it goes from about 30g net carbs to 2.

Basically, any other item on the breakfast menu would follow the same rules: take out bread and sauces and stay away from the hash browns!

Burgers/Sandwiches: Again, follow these simple rules: no bread or condiments (except for mustard), get them wrapped in lettuce instead. All the meats (as long as they're dry) have 0g net carbs and almost all of the toppings have 0-1g net carbs. Absolutely no fries!

Some good low carb options are:

Big Mac (dry no buns): 6g net carbs

Quarter Pounder w/ Cheese (dry, no buns): 7g net carbs

Bacon Clubhouse Burger (dry, no buns): 8g net carbs

Grilled Chicken (dry, no bun): 2g net carbs

Filet-o-Fish (dry, no bun): splurge w/ cheese a side of tartar sauce comes to about 10g net carbs

Salads

Side Salads (no dressing): 2g net carbs

Caesar w/ Grilled Chicken (no croutons): 9g net carbs

Bacon Ranch w/ Grilled Chicken: 6g net carbs

Dressing Packets

Creamy Caesar: 4g net carbs

Low Fat Balsamic Vinaigrette: 6g net carbs

Ranch: 2-4g net carbs

Taco Bell

Taco Bell doesn't have a specifically low-carb menu either, but here are some options for making some of the regular menu items keto friendly. If you're stressing and feel like you just can't find anything, simply removing beans, potatoes, and rice from dishes will dramatically reduce carbs. All hot sauces are 0g net carbs.

Breakfast

Mini Skillet Bowl- with eggs, pico de gallo and nacho cheese (hold the potatoes): 3g net carbs

Power Menu Bowls

Steak Power Bowl (hold beans and rice): 1g net carbs

Ground Beef Power Bowl (hold beans and rice): 7g net carbs

Chicken Power Bowl (hold beans and rice): 5g net carbs

Add-Ons (all 0-2g net carbs)

Steak: 1g net carb

Fire Grilled Chicken: 0g net carbs

Shredded Chicken: 1g net carbs

Seasoned Ground Beef: 1g net carbs

Guacamole: 1,5g net carbs

Bacon: 0g net carbs

Shredded Cheddar: 0g net carbs

Sausage Crumbles: 0g net carbs

Shredded 3 Cheese Blend: 0g net carbs

Sour Cream: 2g net carbs

Extra Cheese Sauce: 2g net carbs

Jalapenos: 0.5g net carbs

Chipotle

Chipotle is a little more health/low-carb friendly than some of the other fast food choices without technically having the options on the menu. They make an effort to keep their ingredients fresh and just about anything on their menu can be made as a salad, which is going to be the best keto option.

For the salad bowls, you can get any of the meats (steak, chicken, pork, barbacoa), cheese, sour cream (make sure it's full fat), red salsa, and guacamole. Steer clear of corn and the green salsas and mix and match all you want!

Sizzler

The buffet side of Sizzler is potentially very dangerous for a keto diet even though it's just a salad bar. There are some very good choices on their menus for keto entrees, but you will have to be careful with the salad bar.

Salads

Asian Chopped Salad (1/2 cup): 3g net carbs

Cucumber Tomato Salad (1/2 cup): 4g net carbs

Greek Salad (1/2 cup): 1g net carbs

Main Dishes

Grilled Salmon w/ Vegetable Medley (6oz, no tartar sauce): 10g net carbs

Italian Herbed Chicken w/ Steamed Broccoli: 9g net carbs

Hibachi Chicken w/ Steamed Broccoli: 12g net carbs (Note: get without sauces and pineapple to bring carb count down)

Shrimp Skewers w/ Cilantro Rice & Steamed Broccoli: 33g net carbs (Note: this is a pretty high carb count! Asking for no rice will bring it down considerably, also request no garlic margarine.)

South Atlantic Red Shrimp Skewers w/ Steamed Broccoli: 42g net carbs (Note: this dish also comes with cilantro rice; no rice will bring carb count down.)

Shrimp Skewers w/ Cilantro Rice and Vegetable Medley: 34g net carbs (Note: another higher carb dish; get it without rice and garlic margarine.)

Tri Tip Steak w/ Vegetable Medley (6oz steak): 8g net carbs

Sides

Tri-Color Quinoa Kale Salad: 13g net carbs (Note: Quinoa is high in protein; if you choose this, make sure you are monitoring protein intake for the rest of the day.)
Steamed Broccoli: 7g net carbs

Vegetable Medley: 8g net carbs

Subway

Obviously, sandwiches are out! But thankfully Subway will make most of their sandwiches as salads that can be tweaked to make them more filling and with the right amount of fat. You can add veggies, usually with no extra charge, or ask for double the meat. You will most likely have to pay for that, but it will make the salads more filling.

Chopped Tuna Salad w/ oil & vinegar (get with extra bacon!): 2g net carbs

Spicy Italian Chopped Salad: 5g net carbs

Cold Cut Combo Salad: 5g net carbs

Subway Club Salad w/ oil & vinegar (double the meat): 5g net carbs

Italian BMT Salad (double the meat): 5g net carbs

Roasted Chicken Patty Salad w/ oil & vinegar: 3g net carbs

Red Robin

If it's burgers you want, the easiest way to keep it Keto is to skip the bun and wrap them in lettuce. Forgo most sauces and condiments or ask for them on the side. You can add bacon for 0g net carbs or cheese for only 1g net carbs.

Wedgie Burger: Red Robin actually does have a specifically low-carb meal on their menu and it's called the Wedgie Burger. It comes on a lettuce wedge and includes bacon, guacamole, tomato, and onion. If you don't want the beef patty you can substitute it with a chicken or turkey burger.

Bottomless Salad: Red Robin is famous for their bottomless fries and thankfully you can swap the fries out for bottomless salad.

Wedge Salad: Their wedge salad is constructed the same way as the Wedgie Burger, just without the burger meat. It is a wedge of iceberg lettuce topped with blue cheese, tomatoes, bacon bits, and onion straws. Skip the onions to make it keto appropriate.

Golden Corral

Buffet style restaurants could make it more difficult to be disciplined. One of the upsides, however, is the fact that you get to fill your own plate. You don't have to feel like you're inconveniencing the servers and chefs. Here are some low-carb meal ideas from Golden Corral. Keep in mind: according to their nutrition facts, quite a few of their dishes contain wheat and soy.

Breakfast: There are not an abundance of keto friendly breakfasts at Golden Corral, but they do have some low-carb breakfast staples you can mix and match to create a meal.

Bacon: 3 pieces= 0g net carbs

Chorizo & Eggs: ½ cup serving= 2g net carbs

Made-To-Order Eggs: 1 egg= 1g net carbs

Sausage: 1 link= 1g net carbs

Meat Dishes: Golden Corral has countless meats prepared in a variety of different ways. Not all of them are keto friendly due to how they're prepared. Here are a few that are good for low-carb diets that don't contain wheat and/or soy.

Garlic Herb Butter Sirloin: 3oz= 1g net carbs

Garlic Parmesan Sirloin: 3oz= 1g net carbs

Lemon Rosemary Sirloin: 3oz= 1g net carbs

Rib Eye: 3oz= 0g net carbs

Boneless Chicken Wings w/ Frank's Hot Sauce: 3 pieces= 0g net carbs

Rotisserie Chicken: 1 piece= 1g net carbs

Baby Back Pork Ribs: 1 rib= 3g net carbs

BBQ Pork: 3oz= 4g net carbs

Grilled Ham Steaks: 2 pieces= 5g net carbs

Seafood: All the seafood dishes contain soy and wheat; it would best to steer clear of those.

Sides: All of the sides either contain wheat and soy or are too high in carbs to be keto friendly.

Vegetables

Steamed Broccoli: ½ cup= 3g net carbs

Steamed Cauliflower: ½ cup= 1g net carbs

Sautéed Spinach: ½ cup= 1g net carbs

Vegetable Trio: ½ cup= 4g net carbs

Dairy Queen

Obviously, the ice cream is off limits. But some of the regular menu favorites can be modified into low-carb options.

Turkey BLT (without ciabatta roll): Sliced turkey, melted Swiss cheese, bacon, lettuce, tomato, and mayo. Hold off on the mayo to bring carbs down even more: 3g net carbs

Original Cheeseburger (without the bun): Beef patty, lettuce, American cheese, pickles, onions and mustard. Only add mayo if you need the extra fat: 3g net carbs

Grilled Chicken BLT Salad: Bacon, chicken, cheese, lettuce, and ranch dressing: without dressing= 7g net carbs, with dressing= 10g net carbs

FlameThrower GrillBurger (without the bun, spicy!): Either one half pound patty or (depending on location) two quarter pound patties, creamy jalapeno sauce, jalapeno bacon, lettuce, sliced jalapeños, tomato, and pepper jack: 4g net carbs

Chicken Bacon Ranch (without ciabatta roll): Chicken breasts, tomato, lettuce, melted Swiss, ranch, and bacon: 5g net carbs

Starbucks (Food Only)

Starbucks has developed a good balance of keeping classic food selections and bringing in new ones. They seem to have focused more on low or reduced fat options, but there are a couple of things that can be eaten on a keto diet. Note: "reduced fat" items are *not* keto options.

Breakfast

Sous Vide Egg Bites: Rich and yummy, these are technically keto friendly but they are on the high end of the carb spectrum, so keep track of carb intake the rest of the day: 9g net carbs per order

Snacks

Snack Boxes: the protein box does include a hard-boiled egg and some cheese, but the rest of the contents aren't keto friendly.

Kind Bars: These are keto friendly, but they are also high in carbs (8g) and they're not even a full meal.

Wingstop

Chicken is definitely a must have for keto diets, but not all forms are healthy. Here are some wing options at Wingstop that are keto friendly. Note: the info listed below is based on an order of 10 wings.

Plain Wings: 0g net carbs

Atomic: 5g net carbs

Mild: 0g net carbs

Garlic Parmesan: 0g net carbs

Cajon: 0g net carbs

Original (hot!): 0g net carbs

Louisiana Rub: 0g net carbs

Lemon Pepper: 0g net carbs

Pair the wings with ranch or blue cheese and celery sticks!

Cheesecake Factory

This chain is absolutely a family favorite! Most of the menu, unfortunately, is not keto friendly but there are a few meals that fit the carb requirements.

Starters: Almost all of the starters are upwards of 30g net carbs and more. The carpaccio is the one option that might have a low enough carb count to work: 11g net carbs (serves 2).

Salads (small options)

Boston House Salad: 11g net carbs

BLT Salad: 15g net carbs

Caesar Salad (with or without chicken): Less than 20g net carbs

Cobb Salad (lunch side): Less than 20g net carbs

Entrees (will have to be modified)

Sandwiches and burgers: order them dry, without the bun/bread

Steak, Seafood, Sides

One option outside of modifying meals on your own is taking advantage of Cheesecake Factory's make-your-own meals. Choose as low carb meats and sides as you can.

Steak Diane: 10g net carbs

Petite Rib Eye: 24g net carbs

Petite Fillet: 23g net carbs

Grilled Salmon: 3g net carbs

Grilled Tuna: 3g net carbs

Grilled Mahi Mahi: 3g net carbs

Herb-Crusted Salmon: 8g net carbs

Green Beans (side): 6g net carbs

Sautéed Spinach (side): 6g net carbs

Asparagus (side): 7g net carbs

Broccoli (side): 9g net carbs

Olive Garden

Italian restaurants can be daunting for any dieter, and there really aren't many low-carb options available. But they do have a few and they even have their own spot on the menu.

Salads & Sides:

Fresh Spinach Salad: 3g net carbs

Oven Roasted Asparagus: 1g net carbs

Bottomless Salad: essentially everything in this salad is keto friendly; even the dressing, up to a certain amount. If you're going that route, ask for a cup of dressing on the side.

Entrees

Herb Grilled Salmon & Broccoli: 1g net carbs

Steak Toscano & Grilled Vegetables: 32g net carbs

Mixed Grill Steak & Chicken Skewers with Grilled Vegetables: 20g net carbs

Alfredo sauce is actually fairly low carb so you can order a side of that for your veggies if you need to make the meal more interesting.

Five Guys Burgers

Five Guys has actually gone out of their way to make their menu low-carb optional, which definitely makes them stand out from the average fast food place. You can literally get any burger on the menu either bunless or in a tin salad-style. You can get the works, all of which are acceptable, except for the ketchup and maybe the mayo unless you need the fat. Here are just a few of the options Five Guys offers. The milkshakes are off limits!

Bunless Hot Dog in a Tin: with relish, onions, and mustard: 7g net carbs

Cheeseburger in a Lettuce Wrap: 1g net carbs

Bunless Bacon Double Cheeseburger in a Tin: try it with jalapeños, bacon, and cheese: 2g net carbs

In-N-Out

In-N-Out has also made an effort to offer low carb choices. They have an entire hidden menu; not all of them are low-carb but a few of them are. Ask for any of the burger protein style to skip the bun and get them wrapped in lettuce.

Double Double Protein Style: two patties, two slices of cheese, special sauce, and all the toppings: 8g net carbs

Cheeseburger Protein Style: single patty, single cheese, special sauce, and all the toppings: 8g net carbs

Hamburger Animal and Protein Style (secret menu): all the burgers can be ordered animal style; it just means the burger is fried in mustard and then they add grilled onions, more pickles, and extra special sauce: 11g net carbs

4x4 Cheeseburger Protein Style (secret menu): four patties, four slices of cheese, two slices of tomato, special sauce: 8g net carbs

3x3 Cheeseburger Protein Style (secret menu): exactly the same as the "quad" but with one less patty, etc.: 8g net carbs

Panera

Although Panera specializes in bread, pastries, and sandwiches, much of their menu can simply be ordered without the bread. They also have a selection of soups and salads that can be keto friendly.

Breakfast: Basically any of their breakfast sandwiches can be ordered without the bread and still function as a satisfying meal.

Ham, Egg, & Cheese Sandwich (without bread): 3g net carbs

Turkey Sausage, Egg White, & Spinach Sandwich (without bread): 2g net carbs

Sausage, Egg, & Cheese Sandwich (without the bread): 3g net carbs

Steak, Egg, & Cheese Bagel Sandwich (without the bagel): 3g net carbs

Lunch & Dinner

Steak & Baby Arugula Sandwich (on lettuce): 10g net carbs

Caesar Chicken Salad (without croutons): 6g net carbs

Green Goddess Cobb Salad (add chicken): 10g net carbs

Italian Sandwich (without bread): ham, sopressa, salami, arugula, provolone, giardiniera, and basil mayo (get the mayo on the side): 4g net carbs

Steak & White Cheddar (without bread): on a bed of lettuce: 7g net carbs

Roasted Turkey & Avocado BLT (without bread): 2g net carbs

Whataburger

Whataburger is yet another burger chain with a menu that can be easily modified into low-carb meals. Here are just a few examples of how to make these burgers keto friendly.

Breakfast

Sausage, Egg, & Cheese Sandwich (without bun): 0g net carbs

Scrambled Eggs & Bacon (3 slices of bacon): 3g net carbs

Sausage, Egg, & Cheese Taquito (no tortilla): 3g net carbs

Lunch & Dinner

Double Meat Whataburger add Double Cheese, Bacon, & Jalapeno (without the bun): 5g net carbs (add a side of ranch for about 1 additional g of net carbs)

Grilled Chicken Melt w/ Lettuce (without the bun): 3g net carbs

Whataburger Patty Melt (without the bun): 2g net carbs

Garden Salad w/ Whatachik'n: 17g net carbs- to reduce carb count, get without the fried chicken and take off tomatoes and carrots. Ranch dressing adds about 1g additional net carb.

Cracker Barrel

This restaurant will forever be a family favorite with its great vibe and scrumptious down home meals. Cracker Barrel has also added some great low carb option to their menu.

Breakfast

Country Grilled Sampler: bacon, sausage, sliced tomatoes, and country ham: 4g net carbs (no toast, drop the tomatoes to lower carb count if needed)

Double Meat Breakfast: three eggs, sausage, bacon, and sliced tomatoes (no toast, drop tomatoes if needed).

Eggs 'n Meat: three eggs, sausage or bacon, and sliced tomatoes: 2 net carbs (no toast, drop tomatoes if needed).

Lunch or Dinner

Grilled Steak Salad: 7g net carbs (not including dressing)

Lemon Pepper Grilled Trout: 0g net carbs (not counting sides)

Half Pound Bacon Cheeseburger (no bun): 3g net carbs (not counting sides)

Grilled Roast Beef: 4g net carbs (not counting sides)

Sides

Blue Cheese Dressing: 2g net carbs

Buttermilk Ranch: 1g net carbs

Spicy Pork Rinds: 1g net carbs

Green Beans: 2g net carbs

Texas Roadhouse

Texas Roadhouse is a very popular steakhouse. Thankfully, with these types of restaurants, the options to order low-carb are fairly plentiful. Between the numerous steak dishes and their choice of salads, staying in ketosis should be a cinch at this restaurant.

Starters

Boneless Buffalo Wings (Hot Sauce): 8g net carbs

Boneless Buffalo Wings (Mild Sauce): 8g net carbs

Texas Red Chili (cup): 7g net carbs
Note: the bowl is considerably higher in carbs; if you are planning on eating an entrée as well, the cup would be the best option.

Salads

California Chicken Salad (meal size): 12g net carbs

Chicken Caesar (meal size, with dressing): 16g net carbs

Grilled Chicken (meal size): 13g net carbs

Grilled Salmon (meal size): 11g net carbs

Caesar (side). 9g net carbs

House Salad (side): 7g net carbs

Dressings

Blue Cheese (2oz): 4g net carbs

Ranch (2oz): 4g net carbs

Caesar (2oz): 4g net carbs

Steak Options (10g and under)

Dallas Filet (6oz): 4g net carbs

Dallas Filet (8oz): 6g net carbs

Ft. Worth Ribeye (10oz, 12oz, 16oz): 0g net carbs

New York/Kansas City Strip (8oz, 12oz): 1g net carbs

Prime Rib (10oz, 12oz): 5g net carbs

Chicken Options (10g and under)

Oven Roasted Half Chicken: 7g net carbs

Portobello Mushroom Chicken: 7g net carbs

Country Dinners (Pork)

Grilled Pork Chops (single): 3g net carbs

Grilled Pork Chops (double): 6g net carbs

Fish

Grilled Salmon (5oz, 8oz): 1g net carbs

Sides

Fresh Vegetables: 7g net carbs

Sautéed Mushrooms: 4g net carbs

Green Beans: 11g net carbs

Red Lobster

Seafood is fairly versatile as well. Many of the dishes are paired with butter sauces, which should be keto friendly. And they have a handy low-carb section on their menu to make ordering easy. And, as heart breaking as it is, you'll have to forgo the classic, addicting cheddar biscuits.

Starters

Buffalo Chicken Wings: 4g net carbs

Shellfish Dishes

Shrimp Your Way (Scampi): 3g net carbs

Wild-Caught Snow Crab Legs: 0g net carbs

Live Maine Lobster (1.25lb, steamed): 0g net carbs

Feasts & Combos

CYO-Garlic Shrimp Scampi: 3g net carbs

CYO- Fresh Wood-Grilled Tilapia: 1g net carbs

CYO- Wood Grilled Sea Scallops: 4g net carbs

CYO- 7oz Wood-Grilled Sirloin: 1g net carbs

Other Fish Dishes

Salmon New Orleans (half or full): 8g net carbs

Wild-Caught Flounder (oven broiled): 1g net carbs

Sides & Salads (under 10g net carbs)

Garden Salad: 9g net carbs

Fresh Asparagus: 2g net carbs

Grilled Shrimp (add to salad): 0g net carbs

Fresh Broccoli: 5g net carbs

Classic Lunch Dishes

Farm-Raised Blackened Catfish: 2g net carbs

Chapter 2: Keto Options at Generic Non-Chain/Mom & Pop Restaurants

Some of the best meals we've ever had have come from quaint little "mom & and pop" restaurants, many of them offering a variety of ethnic foods. They may not be big chain franchises but they make up for it with nostalgia and good food. One of the negatives of these dining establishments is that nutrition details will probably be much harder to come by. There are still plenty of options for making meals low-carb, they just won't be as easily accessible on the menu. If you find you are having trouble putting together a low-carb meal, it's never wrong to politely ask an establishment how some of their menu items are prepared. Here are some tips on how to make some of these ethnic and generic restaurant foods more keto friendly.

Italian

Whenever we think "Italian food", we immediately imagine pasta, bread, pizza, cheese, more bread…so, essentially, carb heaven! Italian food is easily a favorite for many people, and initially, it may seem that low-carb choices will be impossible to find. Thankfully, that is not the case.

Pasta and pizza are very much staples in Italian food restaurants here in America and a big part of these dishes are the toppings, which usually consist of good meats and healthy veggies. Try ordering a pasta or pizza meal but ask for the toppings to go over lettuce. If you can, make sure the vegetables are cooked in olive oil, or even butter, if it's full fat. Grass fed is preferable but not always attainable. Opt for straight olive oil and vinegar for the dressing, unless you've confirmed that their ranch or Caesar does not have excess amounts of sugar, especially if it's house-made.

Grilled chicken, beef, or fish will also most likely be on the menu, you'll just have to forgo carb-loaded sides and sauces. Pesto is an option to spread over chicken but use sparingly because of the pine nuts.

Antipasto ("before meal") platters are often available for appetizers. These plates usually consist of meats, vegetables, and sometimes seafood, all of which are excellent low-carb options.

Soups can be a good keto meal as well, as long as they are made with thinner broths rather than thicker "chowder" bases. Chowders often need starch and/or flour to make them thicken which will knock you out of ketosis very quickly. Steer clear of soups with pasta, beans, or gnocchi in them as well.

Mexican

Mexican cuisine is delicious and exciting, but much of it includes beans and rice in a variety of forms witch is not conducive to staying in ketosis. Requesting meals without the rice and beans will immediately lower the carb count.

You can get just about any meal that comes in a tortilla either on the side or over a bed of shredded lettuce. Cheese, full fat sour cream, red salsas, and avocado are all keto approved. Watch out for the additives in guacamole. If you would rather have that over plain avocado slices, be sure to ask what the ingredients are.

Any meat that is grilled is fine and you can even request it over fajita-grilled vegetables rather than inside of a tortilla. Sides such as ceviche and pico de gallo are also options for spicing up your modified meal.

Japanese/Sushi

A lot of Japanese and sushi dishes already cater to low-carb diets with little to no modification. Granted, sushi does come with rice so sashimi is a better choice. Avoid edamame as well; ½ a cup of those little guys easily reaches 9-10g net carbs!

Miso soup is a good low-carb choice. It is a good keto friendly starter and will help fill you up if you find you have limited keto options. Some Japanese restaurants have a dish called Konjac Ramen, which is one of the few noodle-type dishes that will be low-carb enough for your diet. The noodles are made out of the root of the elephant yam and the single serving size only comes to about 2-3g net carbs. Granted, there are other toppings on ramen bowls, so you will have to be conscientious about the other ingredients to keep it low carb.

As with the other restaurants, grilled meats are always a good choice provided they are not covered in any kind of sauce. Non-seafood options at sushi restaurants often consist of either beef or chicken teriyaki bowls. You could modify these by getting the sauce on the side and forgoing the rice.

Indian

Indian cuisine might be a bit more difficult to get low-carb options for. While the spices are very good, many of the dishes come with sauces and unless you're making it yourself, it could be difficult to find any without sugars or flours used to thicken them. Try to order meat dishes, with little to no sauce if possible, and always skip the naan and rice.

Tandoori chicken can be a good choice; just keep in mind tandoori marinade usually contains yogurt, a lot of which is not very low-carb. Also, any kind of kabobs with meat and veggies are good as long as the meat is dry.

BBQ

Once of the biggest carb hang-ups, you'll come across at a BBQ joint is the sauces. Asking for your baby back ribs with no sauce does seem like it defeats the purpose. But BBQ restaurants are all about the smoking and the seasoning as well. A well-seasoned dry rubbed steak or rack of ribs will be just as enjoyable without the sauce. If asking for no sauce seems like a big deal you can always request it on the side. Sadly, just about every version of a BBQ sauce will be off limits due to the high amount of sugar, even in house-made sauces.

Also try to avoid pre-sauced dishes like pulled pork, barbacoa, or other shredded meats that are prepared in the sauce. Some southern BBQ places might use a sauce made with vinegar and mustard, which will be keto friendly.

If you're ordering wings, ask if there is a dry rub version (like they offer at Buffalo Wild Wings) or simply get them dry with buffalo sauce on the side. Pair them with ranch or blue cheese and celery sticks (try to avoid starchy carrots).

The same salad and side rules apply here as any other restaurant; steer clear of sweet, fruity dressings, hold the croutons, no bread or fried sides!

Sports Bars

Sports bars will probably have similar choices to chains like Applebee's, Chili's, and Buffalo Wild Wings, with the exception of limited nutrition facts and a few low carb choices on the menus. Still, the same concepts work for these non-chain restaurants.

If you're hanging with friends watching the big game, it's easy to just start munching on whatever lands on the table while you watch. Order all of your own appetizers and entrees rather than sharing orders with others who don't have the same diet requirements.

Steak is always a win, which will mostly likely be one of the options on the menu at a sports bar. The same goes for chicken, as long as it's not breaded. Grilled fish, pork chops, and bunless burgers are wise choices as well. Again, be mindful of sides and swap out dippable veggies like cucumbers and celery for the fries or potatoes.

Chapter 3: Keto Options at Convenience Stores & Gas Stations

Let's face it...we all need vacations in our lives! Figuring out what to eat once you're at your destination is one problem. What to eat along the way is another. Any long road trip or even time spent in an airport is going to require a pit stop of some kind. These stops are usually at stores with nothing but chips and candy...or so it seems. Even if there is no road trip involved, a quick trip to a 7/11 store to satisfy the "munchies" could be dangerous ground. Here are some quick, easy, and Keto friendly finds.

Cheese

Yes, cheese is our friend; and a very low-carb, fulfilling snack for on the go. You can get mozzarella string cheese or even jack or cheddar cheeses that come in a similar form. Make sure they are full fat and limit yourself to one or two to keep carbs down.

Raw Vegetables

Many convenience and gas station stores have small refrigerated sections where you can find great keto options, like raw veggies. Try to pick celery or broccoli over carrots and get a ranch dressing packet to go with it. Steer clear of peanut butter and hummus.

Hard Boiled Eggs

Perhaps not every convenience store will have these, but bigger ones like Walgreens or 7/11 might. These are the perfect keto snack and if the egg isn't enough you could even pair it with the veggies.

Cold Cuts

You might also find some cold cuts in the refrigerated section. Take care to read the ingredients, however. Some may be packed with sugary or really high sodium extras. These would also go well with the veggies and boiled eggs.

Jerky

Jerky is definitely an American staple! It is a great source of protein, and you can find it literally anywhere. Poultry jerkies will have less fat than beef, so go with the beef if you need to up your fat intake. Look at the ingredients before you buy it to make sure there aren't any added sugars and get original rather than flavored, like teriyaki.

Pork Rinds

These suckers have been around forever and have taken the keto world by storm! These are an excellent choice if you just need something to munch and you can even dip them in ranch or blue cheese if you need to.

Kale Chips

Kale chips are a fairly new addition to the convenience store roster and not every establishment will have them. If you find a store along the way that sells them, you might want to stock up for the rest of your trip. They are also an excellent substitute for chips or pretzels and can effectively satisfy the need to munch.

Hot Dogs

Any convenience store and most gas station stores will have a hot food section, with items like burritos, burgers, and hot dogs. The burgers will probably come already in the bun but the dogs are usually kept hot on their own. Grab one or two, skip the bun, add some mustard or ranch, and you have a Keto snack to go along with your veggies or kale chips.

Chapter 4: Keto Options: Low Carb Alcoholic & Coffee Beverages

For some, giving up alcohol or coffee may not be so bad. For others, it would be the end of the world! Have no fear; there are easily accessible low-carb options both at restaurants and coffee shops.

Keto Friendly Alcoholic Options

Wine & Beer: If you have to choose between one or the other, wines and champagnes have much fewer carbs than beer. Plus, beer is wheat based which will take your body out of ketosis very quickly.

For a keto diet, even if you're trying to stay below 20g net carbs a day, a glass of wine somewhat regularly would be alright. Try to choose dry wines as they will contain 0.5g sugar and under per glass. Definitely avoid ports and other sweet dessert wines. If there is not a suitable wine choice at the restaurant you might have to search for an alternative.

Beer is basically off limits period if you're trying to stay in ketosis unless you order very light American beers. But if you absolutely need a beer and the restaurant has very low carb choices, then you can safely have one *on occasion* if needed.

Spirits: Straight spirits are all 0g net carbs. It's the stuff that gets added to them you have to watch out for. For example, a vodka and soda water (aka "skinny bitch") is 0g net carbs while a Bloody Mary with vodka is 7g. When ordering mixed cocktails, avoid the ones with added sugars from syrups, sodas, and liqueurs. Dry martinis are also low-carb

Wine Coolers & Alcopops: all of these are off limits for keto diets. They are loaded with sugar; you're basically drinking a soda with some alcohol in it.

Keto Friendly Coffee Beverages

We all have that one friend who you would never want to meet in a dark alley on a caffeine rage. Or maybe you are that friend! Coffee is a staple for many to live through the day and it is very easy to find keto approved coffee beverages.

Starbucks Keto Drinks

Starbucks is probably the most well-known and widespread coffee chain in the world. They may not have too much going on for low-carb meals, but their keto coffee choices are quite vast and delicious.
Black Coffee: This one is kind of a no-brainer; if you want your coffee as low-carb as possibly, drink it black! Americanos are very low-carb as well.

Low-Carb Mocha: Replace the milk in the regular mocha with half water and half heavy cream. Ask for the skinny mocha sauce instead of regular.

Low-Carb Flat White: Replace steamed milk with half water, half heavy cream and you will maintain the creamy texture while cutting out much of the carbs.

Low-Carb Misto: Replace the milk with half and half water/heavy cream. Order it "short" and it will have only 5g net carbs (without modifications).

Low-Carb Vanilla Latte: Replace the milk with water/heavy cream and ask for sugar-free vanilla syrup.

Obviously, Starbucks is a coffee shop and can afford to be versatile. Ordering keto friendly coffee in fast food or sit down restaurants may be more difficult. When in doubt, always order it in black. If you have the option, get heavy cream instead of creamer. Or, you can bring your own MCT oil if it's the fatty taste you're craving.

Use the Starbucks guidelines for ordering espresso drinks at other establishments and beware of the syrups! If you have to have the syrup make sure it's always sugar free and you have substituted the milk for heavy cream.

Side note: all teas without honey or sugar are low carb, so knock yourself out!

Chapter 5: Keto Imposters & "Contraband"

If you feel like you have been sticking to the diet but are failing to see results, you may have been consuming "hidden" carbs and might have dropped out of ketosis.

Keto Imposters

There are the obvious slip-ups in sodas and candy. But even some reportedly healthy foods are not keto friendly at all. Cereals are some of the biggest imposters: 1 cup of cheerios has 17g net carbs, 1 cup of GoLean Crunch has 22g net carbs, Special K has 22g, and shredded wheat has a whopping 39g net carbs in a 1 cup serving!

Health or protein bars can also hide carbs. The chocolate chip Clif Bar alone has 41g net carbs! That's almost double the number of carbs in 1 serving that you should be eating in all your meals for one day on the keto diet.

Many Keto diet shopping lists include some fruits and nuts. In reality, most if not all should be avoided while trying to stay in ketosis. They are just too high in carbs to compensate for the fats and proteins they might be able to offer. The same goes for beans and legumes. If you have to have fruit in your life, choose low sugar berries such as blackberries, raspberries, or blueberries (try to keep serving sizes at ½ a cup or under).

Vegetables are definitely on the list, but not every vegetable is created equal. Take care limit and/or avoid starchy veggies such as sweet potatoes, regular potatoes, corn, carrots, peas, and even cherry tomatoes.

Sugars are an obvious no-no, but they often creep up even in foods we thought were healthy and keto friendly. Even "healthy" sugars can kick your body out of ketosis. Pay close attention to nutrition facts and try to avoid even natural sugars found in honey, syrups, raw sugar, agave nectar, and cane sugar.

Dairy is listed on Keto diets but still should be consumed in moderation and always full fat. Some dairy products that are not actually keto friendly are: low fat or 2% milks, low fat cottage cheese, pre-packaged shredded cheeses (which often include potato starch), low fat or substitute butters, and yogurts (both low and full fat as it is really hard to find low carb/sugar yogurts).

Keto Contraband

The keto diet could be described as fairly easy in, very easy out. In other words, it's not too difficult to go into ketosis (usually depending on what method you use) but it also doesn't take much to go out of it again. Part of making a lifestyle change includes kicking bad habits and cutting out bad foods...sometimes forever. The Keto diet may be temporarily based on your goals and health needs, and some foods may be "borderline" contraband. But if you're trying to remain in ketosis for any extended amount of time without having to start the process over, here are some foods to avoid at all costs in order to stay on track.

Some of the obvious ones that will kick your body out of ketosis are potatoes, all bread and grains (including pasta, even whole wheat), rice, beer, sodas, and juice, low fat dairy products, and yogurt.

Any coffee additives that are artificial (like creamers and sugars) should be avoided as well as cheese spread and some salad dressings. Many commercially made dressings, even potentially keto approved ones, have tons of added sugars. Steer clear of any fruit based dressings (such as berry vinaigrettes) and especially any labeled "low" or "reduced" fat; it's the fat you want, just not the carbs.

Most types of gravy and sauces are flour based to make them thicker and have added sugars for flavors. Finding any that are specifically low-carb at restaurants will be practically impossible, so it's best to always skip sauces and gravy when eating out if you want to stay in ketosis.

As we discussed earlier, there are a very few choices of fruit that are Keto friendly. Most of them should be avoided at all costs, due to their very high carb counts. These include Apples, kiwis, cherries, grapes, bananas, mangos, and citrus fruits.

Desserts that are sugary and/or bread and wheat based are also naturally off limits, such as candy and chocolate (unless it's at least 70% dark cacao), donuts, cakes, muffins, cupcakes, cake pops, and ice cream (unless it's specifically Keto friendly).

Chapter 6: Helpful Tips & Guidelines

One of the many perks of the Keto diet is, it has very few rules. There are so many foods you can eat (that taste great) and it fits perfectly into just about any exercise or training routine. That being said, there are some general easy-to-follow rules that will help you keep your body in ketosis when ordering food on the go.

Meats, Cheese, & Veggies

When in doubt, keep it simple! You won't always be able to quickly find pertinent nutrition facts at a restaurant, so sticking to these basics will keep you safe. Get your meat without sauces, especially if you can't find out if they have added sugars or not. Natural cheeses are preferable over American cheese, but either is fine. Ask for your veggies to be sautéed in butter if you don't like them steamed. Granted, this request may not fly at every dining spot, but many restaurants are happy to accommodate.

No Buns!

Bread is a sure way to carb load too much and knock your body out of ketosis. Even whole grains have a lot of sugar binding lectins in them. *If* you absolutely have to have bread and the restaurant can provide it, go with sprouted grains. But, the easiest option here is really to request the sandwich or burger wrapped in lettuce or served salad-style. Add-ons such as bacon or avocado will help satisfy you and ease the loss of the bread. Many sauces and condiments are keto appropriate; just make sure to keep an eye on the sugar content!

If ordering a salad (whether it started that way or you're creating your own) make sure to take into account *all* of the ingredients! Just because it's a salad, it doesn't mean you're always in the clear. Many salads come with croutons, nuts, or fruit, and high carb dressings. Even some leafy greens are higher in carbs. Go for salads that have meat in them to ensure you are getting enough fats and protein and when in doubt, get the dressing on the side. Greek restaurants are a good place to find delicious low-carb gyro-style salads. Skip all croutons and other carby/sugary ingredients and toppings.

Skip the Breading

The same concept for skipping buns goes for breading on fried foods as well if the breading is wheat based. If you really want what's underneath the breading, it's usually pretty easy to peel it off. You can then pair it with a fatty sauce like ranch or buffalo sauce. Or, you might even be able to order the dish without the breading (chicken wings, for example). There are keto-friendly breading options, such as crushed pork rinds, low-carb breadcrumbs, and parmesan and seasonings, but these types of breading will probably be difficult to impossible to find on a menu or even as a special request. It's always nice when the restaurant is accommodating, but we have to remember to not take it too far.

Watch Out for Condiments

Like we mentioned above, a vast majority of condiments and sauces are loaded with sugars and possibly even an overabundance of sodium (too much of a good thing and all that). Still, it is possible to use condiments and sauces to add flavor without getting into trouble. Any sweet-tasting sauces or dressings (like Teriyaki sauces or BBQ sauce) definitely have too much sugar for keto diets. Stick to fattier dressing and sauces like ranch (dressing or dip), buffalo sauce, sour cream (full fat), blue cheese, and Caesar. Keep in mind, some Caesar dressings are more sugary than others, so keep an eye on nutrition facts if possible. Plain yellow mustard is also a keto safe condiment and you could even ask for sides of butter if needed to get your daily fat intake up.

Making Special Requests

For some, the thought of being "that person" makes us squirm. But, at the end of the day, you have a responsibility to take care of yourself and as long as you keep requests respectful and attainable, you should have relatively little pushback. You should prepare yourself for some discomfort, but don't let that interfere with your health goals.

It's pretty standard these days to request burgers at fast food places without the bun; some joints even have these options on the main menu. Nutrition facts are also now readily available at any restaurant making it easier to quickly customize meal choices. You're more likely to get confused or irritated responses from employees for special requests made at fast food restaurants, so try to keep these as simple as possible. Asking for a burger "protein style" or lettuce wrapped is common enough. Don't give a long list of what you want or don't want; ask for cheese if you want cheese, specify toppings, then just get it dry. You can most likely get ranch and/or mustard easily enough on the side when you pick up your order. Be prepared for screw-ups on fast food special orders…it's just how it goes…and be grateful when they do get it right!

At sit down restaurants, you will be able to request more sophisticated alterations. It's actually pretty common to ask for no added salt to your meal and most sit down and family restaurants (chains especially) now have lite or low-carb sections in their menus. Those options make it much easier to get Keto appropriate meals without having to make special requests. Still, it is important to pay attention to additives listed in nutrition facts and sides that come with a meal. A grilled chicken dish is always a good low-carb choice. If it comes with steamed or even sautéed veggies, as long as butter or olive oil is used. However, these dishes are often served with rice, potatoes, and/or bread as well, which are definitely not Keto friendly. The a la carte options on menus could solve this problem well; you could always add a house salad to make the meal more complete. Keep in mind, however, this could also be a more expensive option. Chances are you could get the meal and opt out of those sides and even ask for double veggies to keep it filling.

Conclusion

Thanks for reading *Keto Diet on the Go*, let's hope it was informative and able to provide you with all of the tools you need to achieve your goals whatever they may be.

The next step is to not be afraid to ask for low-carb options and to try new things. There are times when we fall into ruts when we start new routines because it's comfortable and easier to handle. Starting and sustaining a keto diet may not take as much discipline as other "fad" diets, but it will lose its appeal and ability to sustain if you let it get boring.

If you find yourself in a position where you have little to no info on the food you are ordering just follow the guidelines: meats, cheese, and vegetables. You can never go wrong with these keto basics and you can literally find them anywhere at any restaurant you go to.

A diet that revolves around fatty foods and still helps you lose weight is revolutionary. The more the world catches on to a healthier mind-set, we may see a rise in dining establishments providing low-carb options on their menus. So have fun with what you've learned and seize every opportunity for culinary adventure!

Finally, if you found this book useful in any way, a review on Amazon is always appreciated!

Keto Meal Prep

How to Save $100 and 4 Hours A Week by Batch Cooking

Introduction

Welcome and thank you for purchasing a copy of *Keto Meal Prep*.

The world we live in today is all about hustling to the next opportunity and bustling through the inevitable daily to-do list. While we are succeeding in our careers and family life, we are failing our health by fueling our bodies with fatty convenience store snacks, and fast food eats loaded with extra sugars and carbs.

Now is not the time to blame yourself but realize that you only have one body in this lifetime and you need to begin treating it like the beautiful temple of life it is! But how does someone who is constantly busy and on-the-go eat healthier? Well, I am glad you asked!

The chapters within this book hold two incredible sources of getting your health back on track into one jam-packed book of valuable information and recipes! Let me introduce you to the ketogenic diet, paired with the awesome convenience and power of meal prepping!

The following chapters will discuss what the ketogenic diet is and how it can help you get your life back on track and feeling your best! But the best part of this book will teach you the basics of meal prepping and how it can drastically change the way you fuel your body; with meal prep, there are no excuses when it comes to choosing healthier meal choices because you already did all the work yourself!

Thanks again for your interest in how meal prepping on the ketogenic diet can change your life! Every effort was made to ensure it is full of as much useful information as possible, please enjoy!

Chapter 1: Brief Overview of the Keto Diet

This is a high-fat diet that this is low in carbs and moderate in protein consumption. The ketogenic is based on the metabolic state that you aim to get your body into, known as *ketosis.*

When your body is successfully in a ketosis state, the liver produces ketones, which become your body's main source of energy. The core of the keto is based around the idea that the human body was created to run better as a fat burner rather than a burner of sugar and carbs for energy. The ketogenic diet reverses the way in which your body functions in a positive manner. This means that it has the power to totally change your perspective on healthy nutrition!

Fat Torch Versus Sugar Burner

When you consume items that are high in carbs, such as that daily morning donut, your body has to create insulin and glucose to break it down:

- *Insulin* is created to help process the glucose in the bloodstream by transporting it throughout the body.

- *Glucose* is a molecule that is easily converted by the body as an energy source.

When glucose is the body's primary source of energy, fats are not needed, which means they are stored, also known as that pesky excess weight you want to rid yourself of. When your body uses all its glucose, your brain signals you to reach for a snack, which is typically unhealthy such as chips or candy.

This is where the ketogenic diet has the power to reverse the effects of unhealthy eating by transforming your body into a fat burner instead of a sugar burner. When you lower your consumption of carbohydrates, your body then tries to find another energy source, which is when your body enters ketosis.

When your body reaches the state of ketosis, fat cells release any water that they had been storing and the fat cells can make an entrance into the bloodstream and go to the liver. This is essentially the goal of the keto diet. Despite popular belief, you cannot enter ketosis by starving your body, but rather by not consuming carbohydrates.

Keto Diet Benefits

- More effective weight loss
- Improved cholesterol levels
- Decrease in insulin levels

- Improved blood sugar levels
- Elimination of diabetes precursors
- Decrease in the development of diseases like Parkinson's and Alzheimer's
- Treatment for cancer and growth of tumors
- Treatment for reducing symptoms of epilepsy
- Healthier skin

Foods to Avoid

- *Sugary foods*: cake, soda, candy, fruit juice, ice cream, etc.

- *Grains and starches*: anything wheat and corn-based produce such as pasta, rice, and cereals

- *Fruit*: most fruits excluding berries

- *Beans and legumes*: peas, lentils, chickpeas, kidney beans, etc.

- *Root vegetables and tubers*: carrots, parsnips, potatoes, etc.

- *Condiments*

- *Unhealthy fats*: vegetable oils, mayonnaise, etc.

- *Alcohol*

- *Anything labeled "sugar-free," "diet," or "low-carb"*: these items contain sugar alcohols that can greatly affect the success of reaching ketosis

Food to Embrace

- *Meat*: red meat, chicken, steak, turkey, sausage, ham, bacon, etc.

- *Fish*: salmon, trout, tuna, and mackerel

- *Cream and butter*: Grass-fed is the best

- *Nuts and seeds*: chia seeds, almonds, pumpkin seeds, walnuts, flaxseeds, etc.

- *Healthy oils*: extra virgin olive, coconut, avocado, etc.

- *Herbs and spices*

- *Low-carb vegetables*: green veggies, tomatoes, avocados, onions, peppers, etc.

Chapter 2: Why You Should Be Meal Prepping

There are many people that aspire to live a healthier lifestyle but have no idea where to start or have no time to spare. Eating healthy is one thing, but following through with your health and fitness goals and staying consistent is challenging.

When you have your hands full navigating life, cooking all our own meals can feel impossible, and the temptations of hitting up a fast food joint seem like an easier option.

If you are ready to reach your fitness goals, stop spending extraordinary amounts of money on junk food, then your new best friend is meal prepping!

What is Meal Prepping?

Meal prepping is planning, preparing, and packaging snacks and meals for the upcoming week with the idea of portion control and clean eating in mind. No right or wrong way happens to meal prep, which makes it a great dieting alternative for busy bees to personalize to fit into their daily schedule.

The goal of meal prepping is to save substantial time slaving away in the kitchen while having access to healthier meal options throughout the week. You simply dedicate time to planning your meals and cooking their components. Besides that, you will become *amazed* at the difference meal prepping will make in your day to day life!

Reasons Why You Should Be Meal Prepping

Effective weight loss

When you plan your meals in advance, you will know what you are putting into your body. A meal prep routine lets you control how many calories you consume, which is essential for weight loss.

Saves money

Despite popular belief, eating healthy doesn't have to be pricey. Purchasing things in bulk and taking advantage of your freezer is the key. You know exactly what to buy instead of purchasing ingredients you don't need. Plus, with meals already made, you will save a _ton_ of money on fast food meals - up to $100 a week in some cases.

Shopping is simpler

Once you plan your week's meals, grocery shopping will be a breeze since you will have a list to stick to instead of wandering around the store.

Learn portion control

Meal prep teaches you how to balance what you put inside your body. When you pack your meals in containers, it keeps you from reaching for more food that you don't need. This is essential if you want to lose weight; meal prepping allows you to control the nutrients and calories you eat.

Less waste

Meal prepping lets you utilize all your ingredients for the week before they go bad! This is a much better alternative than trashing expensive produce before you have a chance to eat it.

Saves time

While you will need to set time aside to prepare your meals, you will end up saving time in the long run. Think about it; how much time do you spend with the fridge open? How much time do you waste making a decision of what to eat just to become a victim of tempting convenience foods? With meal prep, meals are prepared ahead of time, requiring you to remove from the fridge and nuke them in the microwave. Easy!

Investment in your health

When you can pick what you are going to stuff your face with ahead of time, you have ample time to make much healthier decisions. The benefits of eating cleaner are endless! Good nutrition is everything, especially if you are looking to fit into that bikini for the summer!

Strengthens willpower

Once you become accustomed to eating healthier, you will find that you no longer crave sugar and carbs. When you have a consistent routine of eating better, you will turn down unhealthy food choices much easier.

Reduces stress

Stress directly impacts your immune system, which can cause you to experience digestive issues, lack of quality sleep, and many more negative side effects. Coming home from work and having a meal ready to eat takes away that everyday stress!

Adds variety to your diet

Once you get the hang of meal prepping, you will feel more confident to try new recipes with new ingredients. Your taste buds will receive a variety of flavor daily.

Chapter 3: How to Avoid the 10 Most Common Meal Prep Mistakes

The way you approach meal prepping will make a world of difference when it comes to successfully implementing it into your everyday life. There are many tips out there regarding choosing recipes, shopping, and bringing it all together to create a week's worth of delicious eats.

However, you need to be aware of the things that could potentially go wrong and be knowledgeable of solutions to avoid meal prep pitfalls.

Mistake 1: Not giving yourself enough time to plan

Meal planning takes time and cannot happen in an hour. When you plan, shop, and prep as soon as you can, you are not giving yourself a sufficient amount of time to process everything, which can make it more of a stressful experience than it has to be.

- **Solution:** Allow yourself ample time to plan meals, especially as a beginner. Set aside 2 to 3 hours per week. Take advantage of the weekend to spread out planning, shopping, and prepping of meals. This will allow prepping to feel like a sustainable task that you can do for months to come. An easy way to do this at first is to make a meal calender for the upcoming week. This will help you plan efficiently and avoid wasting food.

Mistake 2: Not choosing the best recipes for your personal needs

To ensure that meal prepping works the best for you and your lifestyle, you need to understand the importance of what your body needs from the recipes you choose. If you pick a bunch of recipes that don't come close to the criteria, you will be hungry and unsatisfied.

- **Solution:** Choose recipes based on the meals you *need*. While this seems obvious, many people overlook this. Create a list of what you want recipes to do for you.

    - Need recipes to be 30 minutes or less?
    - Are you a vegetarian?
    - What ingredients do you have that need to be used?

Mistake 3: Being unrealistic and too ambitious

Meal planning should be viewed as a marathon, not a sprint to the finish. You will feel super inspired at the start of your meal prep journey, but once you start to get into the depths of planning, you can become easily overwhelmed. You need to ensure that your prep schedule matches your regular schedule so that you can sustain it.

- *Solution:* Begin by creating defined goals and assessing your daily routine and schedule; this will help you to find what is realistic for *you*. Start small and start prepping two to three nights per week. This will give you the opportunity to figure out what works and what doesn't and allows you to tweak it to your liking.

Mistake 4: Not stocking the pantry

Experienced meal planners know how essential it is to always have meal basics on hand. If you fail to keep a good supply of staple items, you will miss all the benefits of meal planning and will likely become susceptible to temptation.

- *Solution:* Stock your pantry with all the basics that you can use time and time again in a variety of recipes:

- Canned goods
- White wine vinegar
- Pepper, salt, and other spices
- Canned tomatoes
- Natural sweeteners (agave, maple, and honey)
- Coconut milk
- Olive oil
- Stock
- Etc.

Even on the days, you feel like you have nothing to consume, those basic components can help you create a yummy frittata, a delicious three-ingredient entre, or a one-pot wonder.

Mistake 5: Not searching for items that need to be used up

Before you head to the store, take an inventory of ingredients you already have in your kitchen and make use of leftover components you have. It's a simple step that helps you to prevent waste and saves you money.

- **Solution:** Before choosing recipes and making a grocery list, look in your cupboards, pantry, and fridge for food that needs to be used first. Turn those greens into a tasty side before going bad or thaw that pack of chicken to create a delicious main course.

Mistake 6: Not jotting down recipes

Meal prepping is all about being organized is you want to be successful. If you fail to save or write down recipes you have enjoyed, you will fall off track and become overwhelmed.

- *Solution:* Stay organized by keeping track of recipes that you have enjoyed and new ones you want to try out. It doesn't have to be fancy; could be a scrap piece of paper or on a whiteboard in your kitchen.

Mistake 7: Not taking inventory before shopping

Once you have picked your recipes for the week, you need to see what items you already have in your pantry. This is a closely tied mistake to not seeing the ingredients that need to be used before going bad.

- *Solution:* Before heading to the store, double check your recipe and the list of ingredients. Check your kitchen to ensure you don't have any of the components already so that you prevent overbuying.

Mistake 8: Skipping pre meal prep

Pre meal prepping is obviously an essential part of meal prep; this is small tasks like organizing ingredients and labelling containers. This gives your future self a giant hand. If you skip it, you are hurting yourself and leaves more work to do on the weekends.

- **Solution:** Set aside 30 minutes to an hour of prep each evening. This will make weekend meal prep a heck of a lot more efficient.

Mistake 9: Trying new recipes each day

I highly encourage you to try new recipes, but it's also important to go about eating a new variety of foods in a strategic way. When you fill up the whole week with brand new recipes, it can become very overwhelming and hard to sustain over a long period of time.

- **Solution:** Don't throw new recipes to the side but build your meal plan around recipes you know and then add 1 or 2 new recipes per week. This will help your taste buds from becoming bored and will also strengthen your recipe collection.

Mistake 10: Failing to have a backup plan

Even the most experienced meal preppers are bound to get stuck at work or have evenings where they are not feeling like consuming the dinner they planned out. Having a plan B is essential to stay the course.

- ***Solution:*** Have a good backup plan and have recipes in your back pocket that you know how to make. These will be very simple and can be made quickly, such as an omelet.

Chapter 4: Delicious Keto Recipes

The following sections withhold a wide array of delicious, easy-to-make keto meal prep recipes that you will certainly want to keep in that back pocket of yours! With these recipes, you will have fewer excuses when it comes to fueling your body in a way that makes you feel better both inside and out!

Breakfast Recipes

Greek Egg Bake

Protein: 15g Fat: 11g Net Carbs: 5g Calories: 175 Fiber: 9g

Ingredients:

- ¼ cup sun-dried tomatoes
- ½ cup feta cheese
- ½ tsp. oregano
- 1 cup chopped kale
- 12 eggs

Instructions:

1. Ensure your oven is preheated to 350 degrees.
2. With the foil, line a baking sheet and with the nonstick spray, spray well.
3. Whisk the eggs and then stir in the oregano, feta cheese, tomatoes, and kale.
4. In the sheet, pour the egg mixture. Then, bake the mixture for 25 minutes.
5. Let it cool and slice.

Can be served right away or kept in the fridge for 4 to 5 days.

Turmeric Scrambled Egg Meal Prep

Protein: 29g Fat: 18g Net Carbs: 6g Calories: 216 Fiber: 11g

Ingredients:

- ½ tsp. dried parsley
- 1 cup steamed broccoli
- 2 tbsps. coconut milk
- 2 tsp. dried turmeric
- 4 eggs
- 8 pre-cooked sausages

Instructions:

1. With the nonstick spray, grease a frying pan and then place it over medium heat setting.
2. Whisk the turmeric, parsley, milk, and eggs together with a pinch of the pepper and salt.
3. In the frying pan, slowly pour the mixture of eggs. Then cook well for 2 to 3 minutes, stirring the mixture constantly to break the eggs apart.
4. Flip the eggs and cook for another couple minutes till you reach the desired texture.
5. Add the eggs to two meal prep containers and add the veggies and sausage to the containers.

Can be refrigerated for up to 5 days.

Three-Ingredient Cauliflower Hash Browns

Protein: 7g Fat: 12g Net Carbs: 3.2g Calories: 164 Fiber: 2g

Ingredients:

- ¼ tsp. cayenne pepper
- 1 egg
- ¼ tsp. garlic powder
- ¾ cup shredded cheddar cheese
- ½ tsp. salt
- 1 head of cauliflower
- 1/8 tsp. pepper

Instructions:

1. Ensure your oven is preheated to 400 degrees. Grease a tray with the nonstick spray.
2. Grate the head of the cauliflower. For 3 minutes, place in the microwave and allow to cool. Ring out excess water with the cheesecloth or paper towels.
3. Place the cauliflower with the remaining ingredients and stir well to combine.
4. On a greased tray, form the mixture into square hash browns.
5. Bake for 15 to 20 minutes.
6. Let it cool for 10 minutes.

7. Serve it warm or place into the meal prep containers.

Can be refrigerated for 4 to 5 days.

Vegan Egg Muffins

Protein: 13g Fat: 9g Net Carbs: 4.1g Calories: 143 Fiber: 6g

Ingredients:

- ¼ cup coconut milk
- ½ thinly sliced sweet onion
- ½ tsp. dried oregano or 1 tsp. fresh oregano
- ¾ cup chopped red bell peppers
- ¾ tsp. sea salt
- 1 ½ cup fresh spinach
- 8-ounce pork breakfast sausage
- 1 tbsp. extra virgin olive oil
- 9 eggs

Instructions:

1. Ensure your oven is preheated to 350 degrees. Grease a muffin tin.
2. Sauté the ground sausage, breaking up as it cooks.
3. When halfway cooked, add a tablespoon of the olive oil, along with the oregano, pepper, and onions. Sauté the mixture till the onions turn into translucent.
4. Cover the pan after adding the spinach. Cook for 30 seconds and then toss the mixture.

Spinach should be wilted. Take the pan off the heat.
5. Mix the eggs in a bowl with the milk, pepper, and salt, whisking till well beaten.
6. To the eggs, add the cooked sausage and veggie mixture and mix till well combined.
7. In a muffin tin, put the mixture evenly.
8. Bake for 18 to 20 minutes.

Refrigerate for up to 4 days and frozen for up to 2 months.

Turkey Chorizo Breakfast Sandwich

Protein: 29g Fat: 11g Net Carbs: 8g Calories: 203 Fiber: 5g

Ingredients:

Turkey Chorizo:

- ¼ tsp. cayenne pepper
- 1 tsp. coriander
- ¼ tsp. dried thyme
- ¼ tsp. cinnamon
- ½ tsp. dried oregano
- ¼ tsp. pepper
- ¼ tsp. onion powder
- 1 tbsp. cumin
- 1 tsp. fennel seeds
- 1 tbsp. paprika
- 1 tsp. sea salt
- 1/8 tsp. cloves, ground
- 1-pound turkey breast, lean ground
- 1 tsp. garlic powder

Breakfast Sandwich:

- ¼ avocado
- 1 cooked turkey chorizo patty

- 1 egg
- 1 whole wheat English muffin

Instructions:

1. *TO make the chorizo:* In a bowl, add the turkey and spices. Mix them well with your clean hands. Create 16 even-sized portions and make them into ¼-inch patties.
2. Cook the chorizo patties in a greased skillet till the patties turn brown.
3. *To make a sandwich:* Spray a skillet and add the egg. Cook to your preference.
4. Toast your English muffin.
5. Serve the muffin topped with one chorizo patty, eggs, and avocado.

Freeze the remaining patties to enjoy throughout the week.

Banana Strawberry Baked Oatmeal

Protein: 14g Fat: 16g Net Carbs: 7g Calories: 154 Fiber: 11g

Ingredients:

- 2 eggs
- ¼ cup pure maple syrup
- ½ tsp. salt
- 1 ½ cup chopped strawberries + more to serve
- 1 tsp. cinnamon
- 2 tsp. vanilla extract
- 3 cups almond milk
- 3 mashed/ripe bananas
- 4 cups oats, old-fashioned
- 1 tsp. baking powder

Instructions:

1. Ensure your oven is preheated to 350 degrees. Grease a baking dish.
2. Whisk the salt, baking powder, cinnamon, vanilla, maple syrup, milk, eggs, and banana together well.
3. Mix in the oats. Gently fold in the strawberries.

4. In the prepared dish, pour the mixture. Then, bake the mixture for 35-40 minutes till the oatmeal sets.
5. Before serving, allow it to sit for 5 minutes. Then, serve the topping with more chopped strawberries.

Leftovers can be refrigerated for 3 days.
Simply reheat the oatmeal with a bit of the almond milk and top with desired fruit if you so choose.

Banana Muffins

Calories: 134 Protein: 11g Net Carbs: 9.8g Fiber: 9g Fat: 4g

Ingredients:

- ¼ tsp. salt
- 1 tsp. vanilla extract
- ½ tsp. baking soda
- ½ cup unsweetened applesauce
- 1 ½ cup ripe bananas
- 3 tbsps. olive oil
- 1 tsp. baking powder
- 1 egg
- 1 1/3 cup wheat flour, whole

Instructions:

1. Ensure your oven is preheated to 375 degrees. Grease a muffin tin well.
2. Light beat the egg and then add the bananas, mashing well. Stir the remaining components, minus the flour.
3. Then add the flour, stirring gently till well combined. DON'T OVERMIX.
4. In the muffin tin, pour the batter.
5. Then, bake the batter for 22 minutes.

Muffins can either be refrigerated for 7 days or frozen for 3 months.

Vanilla Cinnamon Protein Bites

Protein: 2g Fat: 9g Net Carbs: 4.2g Calories: 112 Fiber: 3g

Ingredients:

- ¼ - 1/3 cup nut butter of choice (the creamier, the better!)
- ¼ - 1/3 cup pure maple syrup
- ¼ cup vanilla protein powder
- ½ cup almond meal
- ½ - 1 tsp. vanilla extract
- ¾ cup quick oats
- 1 tbsp. cinnamon

Instructions:

1. Grind the oats in your food processor and pour them into a mixing bowl. Add the nut butter, cinnamon, protein powder, and almond meal to the bowl, stirring well.
2. Pour in the vanilla and syrup, combining well with your clean hands.
3. With the parchment paper, like a cookie sheet, roll the mixture making 1 ½-inch balls and place on the lined sheet.
4. Freeze for 20 to 30 minutes and then place in a Ziploc baggie.

5. Dust the balls with the vanilla protein and cinnamon.

Can be refrigerated for 3 weeks or frozen for up to 6 months.

Low-Carb Breakfast Pizza

Protein: 19g Fat: 16g Net Carbs: 7.2g Calories: 307 Fiber: 5g

Ingredients:

- ¼ tsp. pepper
- ½ cup heavy cream
- ½ tsp. salt
- 1 cup shredded cheese of choice
- 12 eggs
- 2 cups sliced peppers
- 8 ounces of sausage

Instructions:

1. Ensure your oven is preheated to 350 degrees.
2. Microwave the peppers for 3 minutes.
3. In a cast iron skillet, brown the sausage. Set to the side.
4. Mix the pepper, salt, cream, and eggs together and place in the skillet.
5. Cook for 5 minutes till the sides begin to become firm.
6. Place the skillet in the oven and back for 15 minutes. Then, remove the skillet from the oven.

7. To the skillet, add the cheese, peppers, and sausage and then for 3 minutes, place it under the broiler.
8. Allow to sit for 5 minutes to cool. Devour right away or split between the meal prep containers.

Can be refrigerated for 5 days or frozen for 60 days.

Blueberry Pancake Bites

Protein: 6g Fat: 13g Net Carbs: 7.5g Calories: 188 Fiber: 4g

Ingredients:

- ½ cup frozen blueberries
- 1/3 – ½ cup water
- ½ tsp. cinnamon
- 1 tsp. baking powder
- ¼ cup melted ghee
- ½ tsp. salt
- ½ cup coconut flour
- ½ tsp. vanilla extract
- 4 eggs

Instructions:

1. Ensure your oven is preheated to 325 degrees. With the butter and coconut oil spray, grease a muffin tin.
2. Mix the vanilla, sweetener, and eggs together until smooth.
3. Stir in the cinnamon, salt, baking powder, melted ghee, and coconut flour, blending till smooth.
4. To the batter, add 1/3 cup of the water and blend once more. The batter should be thick.

5. Among the muffin tin cups, divide the batter and then add a few blueberries to each muffin.
6. For 20 to 25 minutes, bake until set.
7. Allow to cool.

Can be kept in a slightly cold place in an airtight container for 8-10 days. Can be frozen for 60-80 days.

Lunch Recipes

Shredded Chicken for Meal Prep

Calories: 115 Sugar: 0g Carbs: 0g Total Fat: 4g Protein: 19g

Ingredients:

- ½ tsp. black peppercorns
- 2 bay leaves
- 2 halved cloves of garlic
- 32 ounces of chicken broth (preferably reduced-sodium)
- 4 ½ - 5 pounds skinned chicken thighs
- 4 parsley stems
- 4 thyme sprigs

Instructions:

1. Put the chicken in your slow cooker.
2. In a double-wrapped cheesecloth, place the peppercorns, garlic, bay leaves, parsley stems, and thyme sprigs. Tie off the cheesecloth and add the filled bouquet to the slow cooker.
3. Pour the broth into your slow cooker over the chicken and wrapped herbs.
4. Cover them and set to cook on low heat setting for 7 to 8 hours.
5. Discard the bouquet.

6. Place the chicken in a bowl and leave the cooking liquids in the cooker.
7. Once some of the chicken has cooled, take out the bones from the meat. Use two forks to shred the chicken, adding reserved cooking liquids while shredding to keep the meat moist.
8. Strain the remaining liquids and use for the future stock if desired.

Can be used in a large variety of meal prep recipes! To make ahead, place 2 cups of stock and chicken in separate containers.

Can be frozen for 3 months and refrigerated for 3 days.

Easy Sheet Pan Roasted Vegetables

Calories: 97 Protein: 2g Carbs: 11g Total Fat: 6g Sugar: 4g

Ingredients:

- 1 tbsp. balsamic vinegar
- ¼ tsp. pepper
- 1 chopped red onion
- 1 tsp. coarse salt
- 2 chopped red bell peppers
- 2 tsp. Italian seasoning
- 3 tbsps. olive oil, extra virgin
- 3 cups cubed butternut squash
- 4 cups broccoli florets

Instructions:

1. Ensure your oven is preheated to 425 degrees.
2. Toss the cubed squash in a tablespoon of the oil and spread out onto a baking tray. Roast for 10 minutes.
3. Toss the pepper, salt, Italian seasoning, onion, bell peppers, and broccoli till coated well.
4. Add the roasted squash to the veggies. Toss well to incorporate. Spread the veggie mixture over two baking trays.
5. Roast for 17 to 20 minutes, making sure to stir around 1-2 times throughout the cooking

process. Vegetables should be tender and browned in areas.
6. Drizzle with the vinegar before eating.

Can be refrigerated for up to 7 days.

Mango Coconut Chicken Bowls

Calories: 482 Sugar: 0g Carbs: 72g Total Fat: 8g Protein: 34g

Ingredients:

- ¼ cup sweetened shredded coconut
- 1 sliced avocado
- 2 cups cooked brown rice
- 4 chicken breasts (sliced lengthwise in half)

Mango marinade:

- 1 tsp. salt
- 2 tbsps. lime juice
- 1 tbsp. Sriracha
- 2 minced garlic cloves
- 1 tbsp. honey
- 2 tbsps. olive oil
- 1 mango

Corn salsa:

- ¼ cup cilantro
- 1 can drained black beans
- ½ diced red pepper
- ¾ tsp. salt
- 1 ½ cup corn
- 1 diced red onion

- 1 tbsp. lime juice

Instructions:

1. Ensure your oven is preheated to 425 degrees.
2. Cook the rice as per the package instructions.
3. In a blender, mix all of the mango marinade ingredients together till combined.
4. Marinate the chicken in half of the mango mixture for 10 minutes.
5. Mix together the corn salsa ingredients.
6. On your baking tray, place the chicken and bake for 15-20 minutes till golden in color.
7. Slice the chicken and place into bowls, along with additional mango sauce, corn salsa, topped with the shredded coconut and cilantro. Place the avocado on top.

Can be chilled in your fridge up to 5 days.

Chicken Tikka Masala Prep Bowls

Calories: 215 Sugar: 2g Carbs: 17g Total Fat: 9g Protein: 21g

Ingredients:

- 1 ½ pounds chicken breasts (cut into 1-inch pieces; boneless, skinless)
- 1 cup brown rice
- 1 diced onion
- ¼ cup cilantro
- 1 tbsp. lemon juice
- 1 tbsp. ginger, grated
- 1/3 cup heavy cream
- 2 tbsps. tomato paste
- 1 cup chicken stock, reduced-sodium
- 2 tbsps. unsalted butter
- 2 tsp. garam masala
- 28-ounce can diced tomatoes
- 2 tsp. chili powder
- 3 minced garlic cloves
- 2 tsp. turmeric

Instructions:

1. Cook the rice in 2 cups of water following the package directions.

2. In a skillet, melt the butter. With the pepper and salt, season the chicken. Then, with the onion, add the chicken to the skillet, cooking for 4 to 5 minutes till golden.
3. Stir in the turmeric, chili powder, garam masala, ginger, and tomato paste, cooking for 1 to 2 minutes as you combine.
4. Pour the chicken stock and tomatoes in. Bring the mixture to a boil.
5. Decrease heat. Then, for 10 minutes, let it simmer, stirring on occasion.
6. Mix in the lemon juice and cream, heating through 1 minute.
7. Spoon the rice and chicken into the meal prep bowls and garnish with the cilantro.

Refrigerated for up to 7 days or frozen for 1 month.

Spinach, Tomato, and Bacon Muffin Tin Quiche

Calories: 96 Carbs: 2g Sugar: 0g Protein: 13g Total Fat: 9g

Ingredients:

- ¼ cup tomatoes, diced
- ½ cup low-fat milk
- ½ tsp. pepper
- ½ cup chopped green onions
- ½ tsp. salt
- 1 ½ cup red-skinned potatoes, diced
- 2-ounces shredded cheese of choice
- 1 ½ cup chopped spinach
- 2 tbsps. extra virgin olive oil
- 3 strips of cooked/chopped bacon
- 8 eggs

Instructions:

1. Ensure your oven is preheated to 325 degrees. Liberally grease a muffin tin.
2. Set over medium heat, warm oil in a pan. To the pan, add some salt and potatoes, stirring for 5 minutes till the potatoes are just cooked. Take it off the heat. Allow to sit and cool for 5 minutes.

3. Whisk the pepper, salt, milk, cheese, and eggs together.
4. Fold in the cooked potatoes, tomatoes, green onion, and spinach to the egg mixture.
5. Pour the egg and veggie mixture evenly in your muffin tin.
6. Bake for 25 minutes till firm to the touch.
7. For 5 minutes, allow to sit.

Can be refrigerated for 3 days and frozen up to a month.

To reheat, remove the plastic wrapper, put a dampened paper towel around it, and then heat in the microwave for 30 to 60 seconds. Enjoy!

Taco Scramble

Calories: 450 Carbs: 24g Sugar: 3g Total Fat: 19g Protein: 46g

Ingredients:

- ¼ cup chopped scallions
- ¼ cup water
- ¼ tsp. adobo seasoning salt
- ½ cup Mexican shredded cheese
- ½ minced onion
- 1 pound lean ground turkey
- 2 tbsps. homemade taco seasoning (Tastier and better for you than the store-bought!)
- 2 tbsps. minced bell pepper
- 4-ounce can tomato sauce
- 8 beaten eggs

Potatoes:

- ½ tsp. garlic powder
- 1 pound red potatoes, quartered
- ¾ tsp. salt
- 4 tsp. olive oil

Homemade taco seasoning:

- 1 tsp. chili powder
- ½ tsp. oregano

- 1 tsp. paprika
- 1 tsp. cumin
- 1 tsp. garlic powder
- 1 tsp. salt

Instructions:

1. Beat the eggs, add the seasoning salt, and fold in the cheese.
2. Ensure your oven is preheated to 425 degrees. Grease a casserole dish.
3. Add the oil, salt, garlic powder, and 1-2 pinches of the pepper to the potatoes. Bake the potatoes for 45 minutes till tender, making sure to stir every 15 minutes.
4. Brown the turkey. Then add the water, tomato sauce, bell pepper, and onion. Stir, simmering for 20 minutes
5. Spray a separate skillet liberally using the cooking spray and add the eggs and ¼ teaspoon of the salt. Scramble for 2 to 3 minutes.
6. When serving, put ¾ cup of the turkey and 2/3 cup of the eggs into a meal prep container or serving bowl. Divide the potatoes among each serving with 1 tablespoon of the cheese and scallions.

Chicken Sausage and Peppers

Calories: 249 Protein: 18g Carbs: 20g Total Fat: 11g Sugar: 11g

Ingredients:

- 1 sweet onion (cut into wedges)
- 2 cups grape tomatoes
- 1 tbsp. oregano
- 1 tbsp. vinegar, balsamic
- 12-ounce package of Italian-flavored cooked chicken sausage
- 1 tbsp. olive oil
- 4 sweet peppers, color of choice (chop into 1-inch pieces)

Instructions:

1. Ensure your oven is preheated to 425 degrees. Liberally grease a baking pan.
2. In the prepared pan, add the tomatoes, onion, and peppers. Drizzle with the vinegar and olive oil and toss. Roast for 30 minutes.
3. Move the roasted veggies to one side of the tray and put the sausage in an empty portion. Roast for another 10 to 15 minutes till the sausage is heated through.
4. Sprinkle with the oregano.

Can be refrigerated for 7 days and frozen for 15 days.

Southwestern Chicken Burrito Bowls

Calories: 301 Sugar: 3g Carbs: 10g Total Fat: 14g Protein: 21g

Ingredients:

- ¼ tsp. cayenne
- ¼ tsp. pepper
- 1 ½ cup canned black beans
- ½ tsp. cumin
- ¾ cup canned corn
- 1 cup grape tomatoes
- 1 cup cooked rice
- 1 tsp. paprika
- 2 cups kale
- 3 cups shredded chicken

Instructions:
1. Prepare the rice according to the package instructions. Mix the pepper, cayenne, cumin, and paprika in with the rice when there are around 5 minutes left to cook the rice.
2. Layer your meal prep containers with the shredded chicken, rice, beans, corn, kale, and tomatoes.
3. Top with the dressing and enjoy it right away or store in the fridge for later enjoyment.

Can be refrigerated for 7-10 days.

Skinny Joes With Tangy Slaw

Calories: 381 Protein: 29g Carbs: 23g Total Fat: 14g Sugar: 4g

Ingredients:

- 1 cup chopped tomatoes
- ½ cup rolled oats
- 1 cup water
- 1 red onion, chop
- 1 green or red bell pepper, chop
- 1 ½ tsp. salt
- 1 grated carrot
- 1 tbsp. Worcestershire sauce
- 1-pound ground beef, lean
- 2 tsp. garlic powder
- 1 tbsp. olive oil
- 4 tbsps. apple cider vinegar
- 4 tbsps. tomato paste

Tangy Slaw:

- ½ chopped red onion
- ½ head cabbage
- 1 tbsp. honey
- 1 tbsp. mustard, Dijon
- 2 grated carrots
- 2 tbsps. apple cider vinegar

Instructions:

1. Press SAUTÉ. Pour the oil into an instant pot and allow to heat for a bit. Add the beef and cook till browned.
2. Push the beef to the side in the pot and add the garlic powder, salt, carrots, peppers, and onions, sautéing for 5 minutes till softened. Then pour in the water, tomato paste, chopped tomatoes, vinegar, and Worcestershire sauce. Mix well to incorporate.
3. When the mixture heats to boiling, toss in the oats. DO NOT STIR.
4. Close the lid. Press HIGH PRESSURE. For 10 minutes, cook the mixture.
5. Perform the natural release. Let it sit for a few minutes covered to allow to thicken.

1. *To make the slaw*, combine the honey, vinegar, and mustard.
2. Add the onions, carrots, and cabbage, tossing with the honey mixture.

Sloppy joe meat can be frozen for up to 3 months and refrigerated for 10 days.

Tangy slaw can be refrigerated for up to 4 days.

Mason Jar Recipes

Asian Chicken Mason Jar Salad

Calories: 524 Sugar: 15g Carbs: 39g Total Fat: 33g Protein: 28g

Ingredients:

- 1 1/3 cup halved snap peas
- 1 cup grated carrots
- 1 cup whole cashews, unsalted
- 1 julienned red pepper
- 2 cups baby spinach, sliced
- 2 cups napa cabbage, sliced
- 1 1/3 cup sliced cucumber
- 2 cups shredded rotisserie chicken
- 2 tbsps. green onions, sliced

Sesame dressing:

- 1 minced garlic clove
- 2 tbsps. rice vinegar
- 1 tbsp. minced ginger
- 1 tbsp. honey
- 1 tsp. sriracha sauce
- 1 tsp. sesame seeds
- 2 tbsps. cilantro
- 1 tbsp. olive oil
- 2 ½ tbsps. sesame oil , toasted
- 3 tbsps. low-sodium soy sauce

- *4 64-ounce mason jars*

Instructions:

1. Whisk the sesame seeds, honey, cilantro, garlic, ginger, sriracha, olive oil, toasted sesame oil, vinegar, and soy sauce together.
2. Toss the spinach and napa cabbage together.
3. Assemble the jars by adding 3 tablespoons of the dressing, 1/3 cup of the snap peas, ¼ cup of the chicken, ¼ cup of the cashews, and a sprinkle of the green onion. Serve it now or place in the fridge. *Salads last 3 to 4 days in the fridge.*

Yogurt and Granola Parfait

Calories: 98 Sugar: 4g Carbs: 2g Total Fat: 4g Protein: 5g

Ingredients:

- 2 cups granola
- 2 cups Greek yogurt (any flavor)
- 4 cups berries

Instructions:

- Layer ½ cup of the granola, ½ cup of the yogurt, and 1 cup of the berries into the jar, continuously layering till you are out of ingredients.

Can be refrigerated for 3 to 4 days.

Zucchini Lasagna

Calories: 114 Sugar: 4g Carbs: 3g Total Fat: 9g Protein: 8g

Ingredients:

- ¼ cup minced parsley
- ½ cup diced onion
- ½ pound lean ground turkey
- ½ tbsp. Italian seasoning
- ½ tbsp. minced garlic
- ½ tsp. oregano
- 1 cup part-skim mozzarella cheese
- 1 egg yolk
- 2 tsp. salt
- 1 tbsp. olive oil
- 2 zucchinis
- 6 tbsps. canned tomato sauce
- 4 tsp. parmesan cheese
- 6 tbsps. crushed tomatoes
- 8 ounces low-fat ricotta cheese

Instructions:

1. Ensure your oven is preheated to 350 degrees.
2. Slice the zucchinis 1/8-inch thick and sprinkle with 1 ½ teaspoon of the salt.
3. Bake for 15-25 minutes till the water is released from edges.

4. Lay the zucchini out on paper towels. Reduce the oven temperature to 325 degrees.
5. In a pan, warm the olive oil. Then pour turkey, garlic, and onion, cooking the meat till cooked through. Season with the seasonings. Set it aside.
6. Mix the crushed tomatoes and tomato sauce together. With the salt and pepper, season.
7. Mix the pepper, salt, egg, and ricotta together as well.
8. Layer half of the sauce between four jars. Then layer the turkey, zucchini noodles, and other ingredients. Parsley and mozzarella should go on top. Seal the jars well.

Can be refrigerated for 3 days.

Berry and Nuts Salad

Calories: 92 Sugar: 3g Carbs: 0.5g Total Fat: 7g Protein: 10g

Ingredients:

- ¼ cup chopped almonds
- ½ cup blackberries
- ½ cup blueberries
- ½ cup strawberries

Zesty Dressing:

- ¼ cup orange juice
- 1 tbsp. honey
- Juice and zest of a lemon
- 2 tbsps. olive oil

Instructions:

1. Whisk the dressing components together till blended.
2. In the mason jar, pour in 2-3 tablespoons of the dressing into the bottom. Then layer the berries, putting the almonds on the top.

Refrigerate for 3 days.

Asian Noodle Salad

Calories: 119 Sugar: 4g Carbs: 1g Total Fat: 5g Protein: 8g

Ingredients:

- ½ cup crunchy rice noodles
- 1 cup cooked/shelled edamame
- 4 green onions, sliced
- 2 carrots, peeled/shredded
- 4 ounces soba noodles

Spicy Peanut Dressing:

- ¼ cup olive oil, extra-virgin
- 4 tsp. vinegar, rice
- 2 tbsps. peanut butter
- 4 tsp. soy sauce
- 4 tsp. sambal

Instructions:

1. Whisk together all dressing components.
2. Pour the dressing into the bottom of the jar. Then layer the noodles, edamame, carrots, green onion, and noodles on top.

Refrigerate up to 4 days.

Mediterranean Salad

Calories: 201 Sugar: 2g Carbs: 2g Total Fat: 4g Protein: 13g

Ingredients:

- 1 cup whole-grain couscous, cooked
- 1 tbsp. olive oil
- 2 ounces crumbles feta cheese
- 4-5 slices artichoke hearts, marinated in olive oil
- 6-10 cherry tomatoes
- Juice of ½ a lemon
- Sea salt
- Sprinkle of dried basil, oregano, and parsley

Instructions:

1. Mix all liquid ingredients together to create a type of the dressing.
2. Pour the dressing into the bottom of the jar. Then add other ingredients to the jar as you see fit.

Refrigerate for up to 3 days.

Feta and Shrimp Cobb Salad

Calories: 192 Sugar: 5g Carbs: 2g Total Fat: 8g Protein: 11g

Ingredients:

- 1 chopped hard-boiled egg
- 1-2 handfuls baby spinach and romaine lettuce
- 1 tbsp. chopped red onion
- 2 chopped slices bacon
- 2 tbsps. avocado
- 2 tbsps. chopped cucumber
- 2 tbsps. crumbled feta cheese
- 6-8 boiled shrimps
- 8 grape tomatoes
- Vinaigrette of choice

Instructions:

1. Pour the vinaigrette into the bottom of the jar.
2. Then layer the veggies, shrimp, bacon, and cheese on top.

Refrigerate for up to 4 days.

BLT Salad

Calories: 205 Sugar: 6g Carbs: 6g Total Fat: 18g Protein: 17g

Ingredients:

- 14 croutons
- 2 cups iceberg lettuce
- 2 cups romaine lettuce
- 2 chopped scallions
- 2 chopped tomatoes
- 4 crumbled slices bacon

Instructions:

1. Whisk all dressing components together.
2. Pour the dressing into the bottom of the jar.
3. Layer the veggies, then the croutons and bacon on top and seal.

Refrigerate for 3 days.

Rainbow Salad

Calories: 109 Sugar: 0g Carbs: 1g Total Fat: 9g Protein: 15g

Ingredients:

- ½ cup raw sunflower seeds
- 1 cup sliced carrots
- 1 cup cucumber, chop
- 1 bell pepper, yellow, chop
- 1 bell pepper, red, chop
- 2 cups chopped red cabbage
- 8 cups assorted salad greens

Balsamic Dressing:

- ¼ cup chopped parsley
- ½ cup white balsamic vinegar
- 2 minced cloves garlic
- Pepper and salt
- 2 tbsps. olive oil

Instructions:
1. Whisk all of the dressing components together.
2. Drain the chickpeas.
3. Pour the dressing into the bottom of the jar. Then layer the veggies and sunflower seeds on top. Seal well.

Can be refrigerated for up to 5 days.

Spinach, Tomato, Mozzarella Salad

Calories: 184 Sugar: 3g Carbs: 3g Total Fat: 12g Protein: 11g

Ingredients:

- 10 cups baby spinach
- 10 ounces fresh mozzarella
- 1-quart grape tomatoes
- 10 tbsps. balsamic vinegar dressing

Instructions:

- Pour the dressing in the bottom of the jar.
- Load the jar with the veggies and then the cheese. Seal well.

Can be refrigerated for up to 3 days.

Dinner Recipes

Chipotle Turkey and Sweet Potato Chili

Calories: 423 Carbs: 39g Total Fat: 18g Sugar: 6g Protein: 28g

Ingredients:

- ¼ - ½ tsp. ground chipotle powder
- 1 cup diced onion
- 1 tsp. oregano, dried
- 1 sweet potato
- 1 tbsp. oil, coconut
- 1 tsp. cumin
- 1-pound ground turkey
- 2 cups chicken broth
- 2 tsp. chili powder
- 28-ounces fire-roasted tomatoes
- 3 minced garlic cloves
- Pepper and salt

Instructions:

1. Warm up the coconut oil over intermediate-extreme warmth.
2. Once the oil begins to simmer, place the turkey in a pan. Cook for 5 minutes, breaking up as it cooks.
3. Toss in the garlic and onions, cooking for 8-10 minutes till the onions turn into translucent.

4. Turn the warmth up to high. Pour in the broth, sweet potato, and tomatoes, along with the seasonings. Bring the mixture up to a boiling point.
5. Turn down the heat to a medium setting and let simmer for 10-15 minutes uncovered. The longer you allow to simmer, the bigger the flavor.

Refrigerate for 7 days and freeze for up to 6 months.

Avocado Bacon Garlic Burger

Calories: 189 Sugar: 1g Carbs: 13g Total Fat: 22g Protein: 27g

Ingredients:

- ½ tsp. pepper
- 1 cup chopped basil
- 1 tsp. salt
- 1-pound grass-fed lean ground beef
- 2 eggs
- 3 minced cloves garlic

Toppings:

- 1 avocado
- 16 pieces of bacon, cooked
- 4 slices red onion

Instructions:

1. Mix all hamburger components till well incorporated.
2. Divide the meat into four patties.
3. In a pan, warm up the olive oil.
4. Then, place the patties, grilling for 4 minutes per side.
5. Make the burgers with the avocado as the bun and other desired toppings.

Chutney Cilantro Meatballs

Calories: 375 Sugar: 3g Carbs: 23g Total Fat: 29g Protein: 35g

Ingredients:

Sauce:

- ½ cup water
- 1 chopped yellow onion
- 2 tbsps. avocado oil
- 28-ounce can crushed tomatoes

Meatballs:

- ½ cup quick-cooking brown rice
- 1 tsp. salt
- 1 tsp. ras el hanout spice blend
- 1 pound ground turkey

Chutney:

- ¼ tsp. cayenne pepper
- 1 bunch cilantro
- 1 green onion
- ¼ tsp. pepper
- 1 tsp. sesame oil, toasted
- 1 tbsp. lemon juice
- ½ tsp. salt

Instructions:

1. To create the sauce, push SAUTÉ and warm up the oil. Sauté the onion for 10 minutes. Then add the water and tomatoes, mixing well as you heat to simmer.
2. To create the meatballs, mix the salt, ra el hanout, rice, and turkey together. Form the mixture into 12 meatballs.
3. Put the meatballs in an even layer in the simmering sauce, spooning a bit of the sauce over the meatballs.
4. Place the lid on, using the PRESSURE RELEASE to seal. Press CANCEL and select POULTRY for 15 minutes.
5. While the meatballs cook, prepare the chutney by combining all chutney ingredients together, grinding them into a paste with the mortar and pestle.
6. Perform the quick release on the meatballs. Serve in the sauce and top with the chutney.

Instant Pot Lamb Shanks

Calories: 338 Sugar: 6g Carbs: 19g Total Fat: 37g Protein: 42g

Ingredients:

- ¼ cup minced Italian parsley
- 1 cup bone broth
- 1 chopped onion
- 1 tbsp. balsamic vinegar
- 1 tsp. fish sauce, red boat
- 1 pound ripe Roma tomatoes
- 1 tbsp. tomato paste
- 2 chopped celery stalks
- 2 tbsps. ghee
- 3 pounds lamb shanks
- 2 chopped carrots
- 3 smashed/peeled garlic cloves
- Pepper and salt

Instructions:

1. Season with the shanks with the pepper and salt.
2. Press SAUTÉ on the instant pot, melt a tablespoon of the ghee. Place the shanks into the pot and sear on all sides for 8-10 minutes.

3. As the lamb browns, chop up the veggies. Take out the lamb from the pot.
4. Lower the heat and add the remaining ghee. To the pot, add the onion, celery, and carrots, seasoning with the pepper and salt.
5. Add the garlic cloves and tomato paste, stirring for at least 60 seconds.
6. Place the shanks back into the pot along with the tomatoes.
7. Pour the balsamic vinegar, fish sauce, and bone broth into the pot.
8. Lock the lid. Press MANUAL and set to cook for 50 minutes. Perform the natural release.
9. Remove the shanks to the plate and top with the sauce.

Cranberry Spice Pot Roast

Calories: 312 Carbs: 13g Total Fat: 29g Sugar: 16g Protein: 54g

Ingredients:

- ¼ cup honey
- ½ cup water
- ½ cup white wine
- 1 cup frozen whole cranberries
- 1 tsp. horseradish powder
- 2 cups bone broth
- 2 peeled garlic cloves
- 2 tbsps. olive oil
- 3 to 4 pounds of beef arm roast
- 3-inch cinnamon stick
- 6 whole cloves

Instructions:

1. Dry the meat with the paper towels. Season liberally with the pepper and salt.
2. Press SAUTÉ on the instant pot. Heat up the oil and place the roast in, browning for 8-10 minutes on all sides. Remove and put to the side.
3. Pour the wine into the instant pot. Using a wooden spoon, from the bottom, scrape the bits. Cook for 4-5 minutes to deglaze.

4. Add the cloves, garlic, cinnamon stick, horseradish powder, honey, water, and cranberries to pot. Cook for 4-5 minutes till the cranberries start to burst open.
5. Place the meat back into the pot. Pour in just enough bone broth to cover the meat.
6. Lock the lid. Press HIGH PRESSURE to cook for 75 minutes.
7. Perform the natural release of the pressure for 15 minutes and then quick release the rest.
8. Place the meat on the serving platter and top with the cranberry sauce.

Garlic Pork and Kale

Calories: 437 Sugar: 11g Carbs: 20g Total Fat: 31g Protein: 49g

Ingredients:

- 1 tsp. minced rosemary
- 1 tbsp. red wine vinegar
- 20-25 whole garlic cloves
- 2 sprigs of thyme
- 1 chopped yellow onion
- 2 tbsps. olive oil
- 2 ½ pound pork shoulder (boneless; cut into 1 ½-inch chunks)
- 2/3 cup red wine, dry
- 2/3 cup chicken broth

Instructions:

1. Season the pork liberally with the pepper and salt.
2. Press SAUTÉ on the instant pot and heat up the olive oil. Working in batches, sear the pork till browned. Remove with the slotted spoon. Discard the fat from the instant pot.
3. Add the thyme and onion to the instant pot, sautéing for 5 minutes. Then add the rosemary and garlic, cooking for 60 seconds.

4. Using a wooden spoon, pour wine in to deglaze the bits from the bottom of the pot.
5. Pour in the broth and add the pork back in. Combine.
6. Lock the lid. Press MANUAL to cook for around 40 minutes. Perform the quick release.
7. Stir in the kale. Press HIGH PRESSURE to cook for another 10 minutes. Perform another quick release.
8. Kale and pork should be nice and tender.

Can freeze up to 3 months.

Lemon Pepper Salmon

Calories: 174 Sugar: 1g Carbs: 29g Total Fat: 11g Sodium: 118mg Protein: 36g

Ingredients:

- ¼ tsp. salt
- ½ thinly sliced lemon
- ½ tsp. pepper
- ¾ cup water
- 1 julienned carrot
- 1 julienned red bell pepper
- 1-pound salmon filet
- 1 julienned zucchini
- 3 tsp. ghee
- Few springs of basil, tarragon, dill, and parsley

Instructions:

1. Pour the herbs and water into the instant pot. Place a trivet into the pot and gently place the salmon onto it.
2. Drizzle the fish with the ghee, pepper, and salt. Cover with slices of the lemon.
3. Lock the lid. Press STEAM to cook for 3 minutes.
4. Julienne your veggies while the salmon cooks.
5. Perform the quick release. Press CANCEL. Remove the rack with the salmon.

6. Discard the herbs. To pot, add veggies. Press SAUTÉ and cook for 1-2 minutes.
7. Serve the salmon with the veggies, along with a teaspoon of the cooking fats if you so choose.

Beef and Broccoli

Calories: 259 Sugar: 2g Carbs: 12g Total Fat: 9g Protein: 28g

Ingredients:

- ¼ tsp. fresh ginger
- 1 tbsp. cooking oil
- 10 to 12-ounce flank steak or sirloin
- 2 minced garlic cloves
- 3 ½ cups broccoli florets
- water

Marinade:

- 1 tsp. cornstarch
- ¼ tsp. dark soy sauce
- ½ tsp. sesame oil
- 1 tsp. soy sauce, low-sodium
- 1/8 tsp. pepper

Sauce:

- ¼ tsp. dark soy sauce
- ½ tsp. dry sherry
- 1 tsp. sesame oil, toasted
- 1 ½ tbsp. oyster flavored sauce
- 1 ½ tsp. soy sauce, low-sodium
- 1/3 cup water, cold

- 2 tsp. cornstarch
- 2 tsp. sugar

Instructions:

1. Mix all marinade ingredients together. Add the beef slices and let them sit for at least 10 minutes.
2. Blanch the broccoli.
3. Combine all sauce ingredients together.
4. Warm the oil in either a pan or wok. Add the beef in a single layer to sear. Pour the garlic and continue cooking the meat till cooked through. Pour the sauce in, constantly stirring till it becomes thickened. Add more water to thin it out if needed. Add the broccoli and stir everything well to coat. Season with the pepper and salt if desired.
5. Sprinkle the sesame seeds and chopped onions if desired.
6. Divide among containers.

Shrimp With Zucchini Noodles

Calories: 119 Sugar: 1g Carbs: 4g Total Fat: 8g Protein: 14g

Ingredients:

- ½ pound shrimp
- 1 tbsp. olive oil
- 4 zucchinis, spiralized

Sauce:

- ¼ cup + 2 tbsps. Thai sweet chili sauce
- ¼ cup + 2 tbsps. light mayo
- ¼ cup + 2 tbsps. plain Greek yogurt
- 1 ½ tsp. sriracha sauce
- 1 ½ tbsp. honey
- 2 tsp. lime juice

Instructions:

1. Cook the shrimp till opaque.
2. Warm up the oil in a pan and add the zucchini till tenderized. Drain and let it rest for 10 minutes.
3. Mix all sauce components together until smooth.

4. Split up the sauce into the containers. Add the zucchini noodles and gently stir to coat well. Add in the shrimp among containers.

Shrimp Taco

Calories: 215 Sugar: 1g Carbs: 3g Total Fat: 15g Protein: 12g

Ingredients:

Spicy Shrimp:

- ¼ tsp. onion powder
- ¼ tsp. salt
- ½ tsp. cumin
- ½ tsp. chili powder
- 1 tbsp. olive oil
- 1 clove garlic, minced
- 20 shrimps

For bowl assembly:

- ½ cup cheddar cheese
- 1 cup black beans
- 1 cup tomatoes
- 1 cup corn
- 1 lime
- 2 tbsps. cilantro

Instructions:

1. Mix all of the shrimp spices together. Add the shrimp, tossing gently to coat. Cover and chill for 10-15 minutes or up to 24 hours.
2. In a skillet, warm the oil and add the shrimp. Cook till cooked thoroughly.
3. To assemble the bowls amongst containers, top with five shrimps, a scoop of tomatoes, beans, corn, and a sprinkle of the cheese and cilantro and a lime wedge.

Refrigerate for up to 14 days.

Lemon Roasted Salmon With Sweet Potatoes and Broccolini

Calories: 223 Sugar: 3g Carbs: 5g Total Fat: 19g Protein: 19g

Ingredients:

- 1/8 tsp. red pepper flakes and thyme
- ¼ tsp. garlic powder
- Pepper and salt
- 2 tbsps. lemon juice
- 1 tbsp. butter
- 12 ounces of wild-caught salmon filets
- 4 cups broccoli florets
- 1-3 tbsps. olive oil
- ½ tsp. cumin
- 2 sweet potatoes, cubed

Instructions:

- Ensure the oven is preheated to 425 degrees. On a sheet pan, place the sweet potatoes on one side and the broccoli on the other. Drizzle both with the oil to the pepper, salt, and cumin and toss. Bake the potatoes for 15 minutes and put the broccoli to the side.
- Mix the pepper, salt, thyme, pepper flakes, garlic powder, lemon juice, and butter together.

Heat for a few seconds in the microwave for the butter to melt.
- With the foil, line a tray, spray, and place the salmon on it. Drizzle the fish with the lemon sauce.
- Remove the potatoes, put the broccoli and salmon on the tray, and put back in the oven for another 12-15 minutes.
- Divide the veggies and fish among containers.

Dessert Recipes

Cinnamon Apples

Calories: 102 Carbs: 4g Total Fat: 3g Sodium: 24mg Sugar: 32g Protein: 13g

Ingredients:

- ½ cup brown sugar
- 1 tbsp. cinnamon
- 2 tbsps. unsalted butter
- ½ cup sugar
- 1/8 tsp. nutmeg
- 3 tbsps. cornstarch
- 6 Granny Smith apples
- Pinch of salt

Instructions:

1. Peel and thinly slice the apples.
2. Pour all ingredients into your instant pot. Stir well to combine.
3. Press MANUAL to cook for 18 minutes. Perform the natural release.
4. Stir up the mixture well and serve!

Refrigerate for 7 days or freeze for 2 months.

Stuffed Peaches

Calories: 237 Sodium: 173mg Carbs: 8g Sugar: 36g Total Fat: 11g Protein: 15g

Ingredients:

- Pinch of sea salt
- ¼ tsp. almond extract
- ½ tsp. cinnamon
- 2 tbsps. butter
- ¼ cup maple syrup
- ¼ cup cassava flour
- 5 peaches
- ½ cup slivered almonds

Instructions:
1. Cut off about ¼ inch from the top of the peaches. Remove the pits and hollow them all out.
2. Mix together the remaining components till crumbly. Pour the crumble mixture into the peaches.
3. Place a steamer basket into the instant pot. Add 2 cups of the water and place the peaches into the basket.
4. Lock the lid, press MANUAL to cook for 3 minutes. Perform the quick release.
5. Remove the peaches and allow to cool for 10 minutes.

Can be refrigerated for 4 days.

Blackberry Curd

Calories: 91 Sugar: 28g Carbs: 2g Total Fat: 0g Sodium: 11mg Protein: 1g

Ingredients:

- 2 tbsps. lemon juice
- 1 cup sugar
- 12 ounces fresh blackberries
- 2 egg yolks
- 2 tbsps. butter

Instructions:

1. Pour the lemon juice, sugar, and blackberries into an instant pot. Lock the lid. Press HIGH PRESSURE to cook for a minute.
2. For 5 minutes, perform the natural pressure release. Then quick release any remaining pressure.
3. Puree the blackberries and remove the seeds as best as you can.
4. Whisk the egg yolks and then add to the hot blackberry puree. Pour it back into the instant pot.
5. Press SAUTÉ and bring to a boil. Stir frequently. Turn off the instant pot and mix in the butter.
6. Pour into the storage container and allow to cool. Chill in the fridge until ready to eat!

Refrigerate for 7 days and freeze for up to 3 months.

Cinnamon Pecan Chia Bars

Calories: 175 Sugar: 9g Carbs: 15g Total Fat: 11g Sodium: 143mg Protein: 12g

Ingredients:

- ¼ cup almond butter
- ½ cup pecan pieces
- ¾ tsp. cinnamon
- 2 tbsps. chia seeds
- 12 Medjool dates, pitted

Instructions:

1. With the parchment paper, line a loaf pan. Allow the excess paper to hang over sides for easier removal later on.
2. In a blender, pour in all recipe components. Process till evenly distributed. The mixture should hold its shape.
3. In a loaf pan, pour mixture in. Firmly press into a block that is ½-inch thick. It will more than likely not take up the whole pan.
4. Chill for 45 minutes till the mixture has set. Slice into the bars.

Chocolate Coconut Bites

Calories: 71 Sugar: 1g Carbs: 21g Total Fat: 16g Sodium: 196mg Protein: 7g

Ingredients:

- ½ cup pecans
- 1 tbsp. cocoa powder
- ½ cup shredded coconut flakes, unsweetened
- 1 tbsp. milk, almond
- 1 tbsp. chia seeds
- 1 tbsp. collagen peptides
- 1 tbsp. liquid coconut oil
- 2 tbsps. hemp seeds
- 8 dates, pitted
- Extra coconut flakes (optional)

Instructions:

1. Blend all recipe components within a food processor till well incorporated.
2. Roll the mixture into 1-inch balls. Roll in additional coconut flakes if you so choose.

Freeze for up to 60 days.

Oatmeal Energy Bites

Calories: 71 Sugar: 1g Carbs: 21g Total Fat: 16g Sodium: 196mg Protein: 7g

Ingredients:

- ½ cup almond butter
- ¼ cup ground flax seed
- 1 cup oats, rolled
- 1/3 cup honey, raw
- ½ cup chocolate chips

Instructions:

1. Mix all recipe components together.
2. Roll out teaspoon-sized balls onto a tray lined with the parchment paper.
3. Freeze the balls for 1 hour.

Freeze for up to 1 month.

Fat Bomb Recipes

Walnut Orange Chocolate Bombs

Calories: 87 Sugar: 1g Carbs: 2g Total Fat: 9g Protein: 2g

Ingredients:

- ¼ cup extra virgin coconut oil
- ½-1 tbsp. orange peel or orange extract
- 1 ¾ cup chopped walnuts
- 1 tsp. cinnamon
- 10-15 drops stevia
- 125 g 85% cocoa dark chocolate

Instructions:

1. Melt the chocolate with your choice of method.
2. Add the cinnamon and coconut oil. Sweeten the mixture with the stevia.
3. Pour in the fresh orange peel and chop the walnuts.
4. In a muffin tin or in the candy cups, spoon in the mixture.
5. Place in the fridge for 1-3 hours until the mixture is solid.

Mini Lemon Tart Bombs

Calories: 101 Protein: 3g Carbs: 1g Total Fat: 11g

Ingredients:

Crust:

- ¾ cup grated dried coconut
- 1 ½ tsp. vanilla extract
- 1 cup almond, cashew or other nut flour
- 2 tbsps. sugar substitute
- 3 tbsps. lemon juice
- 4 ½ tbsps. melted ghee
- Pinch of salt

Filling:

- ¼ tsp. salt
- 1/3 cup lemon juice
- ½ cup softened butter or ghee
- 1 tbsp. sugar substitute
- 1/3 cup full-fat almond or coconut milk
- zest of 2 lemons
- 1 tsp. sugar-free vanilla extract
- 2 tsp. lemon extract

Instructions:

1. *For the crust:* Combine entirely crust ingredients in a medium-sized bowl together. Then roll into a log shape with the help of the waxed paper.
2. Proceed to cut into 20-24 slices.
3. Roll each slice into a ball and press gently into the tart pans.
4. Chill until you are ready to fill the crusts.

5. *For the filling:* In a food processor, pour in the butter and beat till fluffy in the texture.
6. Add the salt, zest, extracts, sweetener, lemon juice, and milk, blending until smooth.
7. Taste the mixture periodically and add more lemon juice or sweetener until it meets your taste bud needs.
8. Then pour the filling into your frozen crusts.
9. Top with a sprinkle of the lemon zest.
10. Chill until the tarts are set. Should make about 24 tarts.

Cinnamon Roll Bomb Bars

Calories: 102 Carbs: 2g Total Fat: 15g Protein: 2g

Ingredients:

- ½ cup creamed coconut
- 1/8 tsp. cinnamon

First icing:

- 1 tbsp. butter, almond
- 1 tbsp. coconut oil, extra-virgin

Second icing:

- ½ tsp. cinnamon
- 1 tbsp. coconut oil (extra virgin) or almond butter

Instructions:

1. With the liners, line a mini loaf pan or baking dish.
2. Using your clean hands, combine the cinnamon and coconut cream. Then pat into a dish.
3. In a separate bowl, mix almond butter and coconut oil together. Then spread the mixture over the creamed coconut.
4. Place in the freezer for 5-10 minutes.

5. In yet another bowl, whisk together ingredients of second icing until combined. Drizzle the icing over bars and let it freeze again for 10-20 minutes.
6. Cut into bars and enjoy!

Can be frozen for up to 3 months.

Macadamia Chocolate Fudge Bombs

Calories: 267 Protein: 3g Carbs: 3g Total Fat: 19g

Ingredients:

- ¼ cup heavy cream or coconut oil
- 2 tbsps. sweetener of choice
- 2 ounces cocoa butter
- 2 tbsps. unsweetened cocoa powder
- 4 ounces chopped macadamias

Instructions:

1. In a saucepan, melt the cocoa butter over a simmering pot of water and then add the cocoa powder. Combine.
2. Pour in the sweetener and macadamia nuts and stir well.
3. Then add the cream, mixing well and bringing the mixture back to room temperature.
4. Pour the mixture into the molds or candy cups. Allow time for the bombs to cool and chill to harden.

Peanut Butter Chocolate Bombs

Calories: 211 Protein: 3.5g Carbs: 2g Total Fat: 15g

Ingredients:

- ¼ cup chopped walnuts
- ½ cup butter or coconut oil
- ½ cup natural peanut butter, plain or chunky
- ½ tsp. vanilla extract
- 1 cup sweetener of choice
- 1/3 cup powder, cocoa
- 2 ounces cream cheese, softened
- 1/3 cup vanilla whey powder
- Dash of salt

Instructions:

1. Line a 5 x 7 dish with the parchment paper, ensuring there is an overhang of paper of two sides to aid in the removal later on. Spread the melted butter over the paper as well.
2. In a saucepan on low heat setting, melt the butter and peanut butter together, combining well.
3. In another bowl, beat the cream cheese until it soft and proceed to beat in the peanut butter until smoothened mixture.
4. Add sugar substitute and vanilla.
5. Mix together the salt, protein powder and cocoa powder in a separate bowl, sifting dry

ingredients into wet ones until smooth in texture. Stir in nuts.
6. Spread the fudge mixture into the prepared pan, placing in the freezer to harden.
7. Remove and cut into squares. Store in the chilled area before serving.

Savory Mediterranean Fat Bombs

Calories: 164 Protein: 4g Carbs: 2g Total Fat: 17g

Ingredients:

- ¼ cup butter or ghee
- ¼ tsp. salt
- ½ cup full-fat cream cheese
- 2 crushed garlic cloves,
- 2-3 tbsps. freshly chopped herbs
- 4 pieces of drained sun-dried tomatoes
- 4 pitted olives
- 5 tbsps. grated parmesan cheese

Instructions:
1. In a bowl, cut butter into tiny pieces. Then add cream cheese.
2. Let it sit in room temperature for 20-30 minutes until soft.
3. Mash together with the fork until mixed. Add the tomatoes and olives.
4. Add the garlic and herbs, and season to taste with the salt and pepper.
5. Mix well ingredients together.
6. Put in the fridge for 20-30 minutes until solidified.
7. Take out the mixture and form five small balls. Then proceed to the roll balls into the grated parmesan cheese.
8. Eat right away or store in the fridge.

Bacon Guac Bombs

Calories: 156 Protein: 5g Carbs: 1g Total Fat: 15g

Ingredients:

- 4 slices of bacon
- ¼ tsp. salt
- 1 tbsp. lime fresh lime juice
- ½ small diced onion
- 1 chopped chili pepper
- 2 cloves crushed garlic
- ¼ cup butter or ghee
- ½ large avocado
- 1-2 tbsps. freshly chopped cilantro
- 1/8 tsp. cayenne pepper

Instructions:

1. Ensure the oven is preheated to 375 degrees.
2. Using the parchment paper, line a baking tray and proceed to lay out the bacon slices, ensuring none overlap.
3. Cook the bacon for 10-15 minutes or until golden brown. Remove and let it cool.
4. In a bowl, mash together the remaining ingredients together until combined. Then add diced onion.

5. Add the bacon grease and combine. Cover the mixture with the foil and put into the fridge for 20-30 minutes.
6. Crumble the bacon to use as breading.
7. Roll the avocado mixture into about six balls and roll into bacon pieces.

Salmon Bombs

Calories: 147 Protein: 3g Carbs: 0.5g Total Fat: 16g

Ingredients:

- ½ cup cream cheese, full-fat
- 1 tbsp. lemon juice, fresh
- ½ package smoked salmon or smoked mackerel
- 1/3 cup butter
- 1-2 tbsps. chopped fresh or dried dill

Instructions:

1. In a food processor, pour in salmon, butter, and cream cheese, adding the lemon juice and dill while pulsing.
2. With the parchment paper, line a tray and place the salmon mixture in 2.5 tablespoon sizes on the tray.
3. Top with the dill and put in the fridge to chill for 1-2 hours until firm.

Jalapeno and Cheese Bombs

Calories: 142 Protein: 4g Carbs: 1g Total Fat: 15g

Ingredients:

- ¼ cup grated cheddar cheese
- ¼ cup unsalted butter
- 2 g halved, seeded, & chopped jalapeño peppers
- 3.5 ounces of full-fat cream cheese
- 4 slices of bacon

Instructions:

1. Ensure your oven is preheated to 325 degrees.
2. With the parchment paper, line a baking sheet, ensuring there is extra hanging over the edge to aid in removing later.
3. Mash together the cream cheese and butter in a bowl and then put in the food processor, mix until smooth in texture.
4. Lay out the bacon slices on the parchment paper, leaving a space between them. Cook for 25-30 minutes until the slices are crispy. Remove and set aside to allow to cool.
5. Add together the cheese and jalapeños to the cream cheese and butter mixture. Chill for half an hour to 1 hour until set.
6. Split up the mixture into six fat bombs and place them on the parchment paper. If serving

right away, roll in the crumbled bacon. If later, chill the mixture before coating in the bacon.

Pizza Bombs

Calories: 112 Protein: 5g Carbs: 2g Total Fat: 10.5g

Ingredients:

- 14 slices of pepperoni
- 2 tbsps. freshly chopped basil
- 2 tbsps. sun-dried tomato pesto
- 4 ounces of cream cheese
- 8 pitted black olives

Instructions:

1. Chop up the olives and pepperoni.
2. In a bowl, mix all together the cream cheese, tomato pesto, and basil and add the pepperoni and olives, mixing well to combine.
3. Form the mixture into balls and then top with the pepperoni, basil, and olive.

Rice Alternatives

One of the toughest challenges when doing keto is finding substitutes for plain old white rice. Here's 10 easy ones.

Cauliflower Rice
Just mince up cauliflower to a rice-like consistency in a food processor and you're good to go. One serving even contains a day's worth of Vitamin C

Broccoli Rice
Same as above - also looks great for photos!

Green Bean Fries
Sauteed green beans with some garlic and olive oil go well with so many different meals.

Zucchini Noodles
A great way to add some more bulk to meals, ideal if you naturally need to eat a higher volume of food to stay full. Use a spiralizer to make these.

Butternut Squash Noodles
Same as above

...and the one food which isn't keto friendly - but everyone thinks is...

Quinoa!
Whether it's red, black or white quinoa, all of these have more than 30g of net carbs per serving, and as such, will usually break your state of ketosis. Avoid quinoa if you're doing keto.

Emergency Keto Meals at Popular Fast Food Chains

As much as we like to plan, it's not possible to stay consistent 100% of the time. Life gets in the way. Fortunately, most fast food chains now have keto friendly meals. Here's a few options at the big chains.

Subway

Skip the bread (duh) and opt for a salad instead. The tuna salad with cheese, black olives, green peppers, lettuce, spinach and pickles has just 330 calories and 7G net carbs. Don't bother with dressings or sauces outside of olive oil, salt and pepper - and you're good to go

Chipotle

A salad bowl with meat, tomato based salsa (no corn), sour cream and cheese is both delicious and keto-approved.

McDonald's

Pro-tip, you can order the sandwiches without bread! Some restaurants might give you a strange look. Worst case scenario you order normally and toss out the bun. The McDouble, McChicken and Grilled Chicken

Sandwich are all keto friendly. As are the sausage and egg mcmuffins

Burger King

Same applies here, a Whopper or Double Cheeseburger without bread or ketchup is keto friendly.

Taco Bell

This one is a little more complicated - order a side of lettuce, side of beef, side of chicken, and side or two of guacamole, then combine for a quick and cheap meal.

KFC

Protein heaven over at the colonel. Grilled chicken thighs are 17g protein with 0 carbs per piece. Breasts are 38g with no carbs. You can also get a side of green beans.

Carl's Jr.

One of the few places which actually has Lettuce-wrapped as an option. The thickburger is just 9G of carbs when you opt for this keto-friendly choice.

Jimmy John's

Any of their sandwiches can be made as Unwiches (order a slim one if you want a save a few bucks) which means no bread.

Five Guys

Same as Carl's Jr. Just order the lettuce wrap options and you're good to go.

In-n-Out

Order your burger "protein style" - a hamburger, cheeseburger or double double comes it at 11G of net carbs with this method.

Chapter 5: Methods to Properly Store Food

Congratulations! So far you know the ins and outs of the ketogenic diet, meal prep mistakes to avoid, and a nice array of keto meal prep recipes to get you started! Now, it's time to discover the proper way to store your deliciously prepped meals so that you can enjoy them as if they were fresh off the press!

Pantry Tips

There are many other items besides fruits, veggies, and canned goods that can reside happily in a pantry. These tips pertain to the foods in storage that don't need to be frozen or refrigerated:

- To lengthen the time of prepper foods, store them in the plastic or glass meal prep containers

- Most canned foods that are low in acid, such as vegetables, crab meat, and tuna can last up to 2 to 5 years. Ensure you check the date.

- Canned foods that are high in acid, like the tomato-based items, pineapple, and grapefruit have a shelf life of 12 to 18 months.

- Conditions of storage areas should be cool, dark, and dry with temperatures that range from 50 to 70 degrees. Warm climate makes the food deteriorate faster, so keep the items away from the hot pipes, dishwasher, and oven.

Fridge Tips

- Stay alert for spoiled food. If anything looks or smells off, it should be thrown out. Yes, mold can happen in the fridge too.

- Keep the prepped meals covered and in the plastic or glass containers, wrapped in the foil or plastic wrap.

- Pay attention to the expiration dates.

- Be vigilant of the 2-hour rule of refrigeration, meaning not leaving items that require to be chilled out for more than 2 hours, such as dairy, seafood, eggs, meat, chicken, etc.

- Set the temperature in your fridge to 40 degrees or lower.

Freezer Tips

I want to nicely remind you that freezing meals does not kill bacteria, but it can stop it from growing. Most frozen foods can last for a long time, but the color, flavor, and tenderness of the frozen items can be affected the longer they are frozen.

- Thaw food in your fridge before prepping

- Don't fear the freezer burn; it's a quality of food issue, not a food safety problem

- Label all packages you freeze with the date, what food is in it, and any other identifying information that will help your meal prep efforts, such as what it weighs or how many servings are in the container

- Ensure that you properly wrap the food you wish to freeze, utilize the airtight storage containers, and use the bags, plastic wrap, and foil that is freezer-grade

- Set the temperature of your freezer to 0 degrees or below

Freezer vs. Fridge

Not all edibles are freezer friendly:

- Fruits high in water content
- Lettuce
- Uncooked batters
- Eggs
- Cooked pasta
- Soft cheeses
- Cultured dairy

Freeze your meals if you don't plan to consume them in 3 to 4 days after you prepare them. Remember that the prepping frozen meals take a bit more preparation time than refrigerated meals.

- Thaw out meals for a few hours or overnight before heating and consuming

- Frozen meals last substantially longer than refrigerated meals, some being able to be frozen up to 1 year

Refrigerated meals are capable of being tasty, fresh, and convenient for a few days. After prepping, you just have to nuke the meals in the microwave. After several days of living in the fridge, however, meals can lose their freshness, taste, and moisture. This is because dry air circulating takes the moisture out of the food. Refrigerate the meals you plan to eat in 3 to 4 days.

Chapter 6: Meal Prep Kitchen Essentials

Setting the time aside each week to prep meals for the entire week is a great way to eliminate the cravings for unhealthy eats and keep you on the right track to achieving your health and fitness goals.

Many people avoid the task of meal planning and prepping simply because they think of it as another chore; this is because they are using the wrong kitchen tools to get this big job done. This chapter will share the essential tools you need to simplify the process of meal prepping and make it more manageable.

High-quality knives

One of the most crucial tools to meal prep is having a decent set of knives that allow you to slice, dice, chop, and chiffonade like a master chef! If you have dull knives in your kitchen drawers, you are *asking* for prepping disaster. Sharp knives will save you time and make meal prep a lot easier on your hands. I recommend stainless steel knives for longevity!

Measuring spoons and cups

If you are meal prepping around macro measurements, it's very crucial to ensure you are measuring correctly. Measuring cups can help you measure dry ingredients like nuts and seeds while measuring spoons will help measure spices.

Food scale

Even though the majority of people can easily get away with measuring with cups and spoons, there are some people that need to ensure accuracy with a food scale. These are also helpful to measure proteins.

Good kitchen utensils

Having good quality kitchen utensils is obviously essential for breezing through meal prep! When you have well-rounded utensils, you can better prepare a variety of meals with ease.

Cutting boards

Almost all meal prep recipes involve dicing, cutting, or chopping, so you need one of these at arm's length always.

Mixing bowls

Good mixing bowls are used to mix batters, marinate proteins, and much more.

Colander

Good for draining veggies and aiming for clean-tasting produce. You want crispy, rainbow-like vegetables, right?

Grater

Meal preppers love graters! It allows them to add lots of flavors to any recipe with a few simple swipes. Zest a lemon, shave some chocolate, grate a bit of nutmeg, etc.

Baking dishes

- Round cake pans
- 13 x 9 baking sheet
- 8 x 8 and 9 x 5 loaf pans
- Muffin pans
- Etc.

Non-stick skillet

Skillets are highly versatile, and you can cook just about anything in them with a little bit of fat.

Cast iron skillet

An amazing gadget for the keto diet, this skillet is capable of adding flavor and iron to your meals.

Sauté pans

Saucepan with lid

Sheet pans

Roasting pan

Cook an amazing evening meal that makes a ton of leftovers! You can even make extremely large batches of items such as granola.

Cooling rack

Spiralizer

Obviously regular pasta is not keto friendly, but a better, healthier alternative can be created with the help of spiralizing vegetables like zucchini. Yum!

Food Processor

Don't want to chop your veggies? Stick them in a food processor! Great for making pesto, hummus, dips, shredding chicken, etc.

Crockpot

Crock pots are a meal prepper's *dream* appliance; if you want to further your meal prep skills, you can save even *more* time with these babies and can make a large variety of meals and desserts.

High-speed blender

No matter if you are making the nut butter, sauces, soups, or smoothies, a good blender is a must and can help you blend in seconds!

Meal prep containers

Quality meal prep containers are an essential staple to the meal planning world. You want ones that are durable and that you can use consistently for a long period of time. Opt for containers with lockable lids rather than the standard lids which can fall off because of condensation.

Made in the USA
San Bernardino, CA
16 June 2019